The Caregiver Zone

By

Judy Castleberry, NHA

Contributions by

Steve Everhart, Certified Senior Advisor (CSA)

Published by

The Senior's Choice
774 Mays Blvd., Suite# 297
Incline Village, NV 89451

The Caregiver Zone

ISBN 0-9760602-0-5

Book design by Pavel Bosak, All Elements Design
Cover design by Pavel Bosak and Caren Parnes
Edited by Caren Parnes, Enterprising Graphics

Printed in the United States of America

TABLE OF CONTENTS

TABLE OF CONTENTS (Continued)

FOREWORD

It has been said "the greatness of a culture can be judged by its heroes." I believe that the family caregivers of the elderly are truly the nation's under-appreciated heroes. As a family caregiver, you deserve all the help and support we can give you. This book is intended to serve as a roadmap for you in your journey through eldercare. We hope to make the road less bumpy for you, your immediate family, and your elderly loved ones. I pray that it is also an inspiration for you to care for yourself first, and to reach out to others who can help.

As a baby boomer with aging parents, and in my rewarding work as founder and president of *The Senior's Choice, Inc.*, a national network of senior care providers, I am intimately aware of the many issues facing seniors and their families. Many of us have faced, or will soon face, the emotional and financial consequences of mom or dad's loss of independence. As we come to terms with these challenges, we are further shocked to learn that neither the family physician nor any other health care professional, has a concise plan for what to do next or where to turn for help.

While there are many books written on the subject of eldercare, none provide you with a clear plan of action. I just could not imagine the already burdened family caregiver finding the time and energy to wade through voluminous chapters looking for things they really need to know and do. Thus, Judy Castleberry and I collaborated on this work to create a concise, practical and enjoyable guide to caring for your elderly loved one.

It is my profound pleasure to be associated with Judy Castleberry of *Partners Assisted Living Services, Inc.* Judy has vast experience in senior care and her focus on clients' individual needs is exemplary. We are proud that she is a fellow member of *The Senior's Choice®*.

We at *The Senior's Choice®* have helped establish and support hundreds of in-home senior companion care companies across North America and we take pride in the standards of excellence common among all our members. Judy's demonstrated character, integrity and love of seniors makes her a savior with her elderly clients and family members, allowing them to enjoy greater independence, peace of mind and the lifestyles they so richly deserve.

Judy has over two decades of experience in eldercare, serving as a nursing home administrator and co-owner of a successful senior companion care company. Combining her personal experience as a daughter of aging parents with her professional experience, Judy has seen all sides of the continuum of eldercare. She really understands what you're going through.

Caring for an elderly adult, regardless of the relationship, requires more than good intentions and love. It takes patience, understanding, and most importantly, knowledge and skills. One person can make a dramatic impact in the life of another, and nowhere is that more evident than in your role as a caregiver. This book was written with you—the family caregiver—in mind. It is meant to be an "easy read" that gives you an accessible caregiving *plan of action* with useful things to do as well as information you need to know.

Your caregiving journey may take you to places you never imagined. In the process you will have the opportunity to learn more about yourself than ever before. Each day may bring life-altering challenges that offer you the opportunity to develop skills and talents you never knew you possessed: resourcefulness, stamina, flexibility, and faith, to name a few. It is unlikely that you will come away from the caregiving experience unchanged.

The simple truth about elders is this: they want their lives to be validated and they do not want to die alone. Go to them as best you can. This is a small price to pay for the riches you will receive in return for doing this work. Eldercare awakens the soul, brings us face-to-face with our own mortality and teaches us to live in the present. Caring for the elderly can serve as a daily reminder of what is ultimately important in our lives. Every privileged conversation that we share with our elderly loved one brings us closer to who we are and makes us wiser in ways that are eventually revealed to us over time.

Steve Everhart
June 3, 2004

PREFACE

When I first started planning this book, I thought of all of those families that I have encountered over my twenty-four years in senior care. This has included long term care facilities, senior apartments, an assisted living facility, a durable medical equipment provider, and most recently, as the co-owner of a companion care agency. Over the years, I have shared a few tears, lots of hugs, a good dose of laughter, and a portion of a lot of folks lives.

Over and over I have heard that one of the biggest problems for many folks is the need for basic information about senior care. That is what this book is all about. My hope is that this little book will be a support to you as you go through one of the most challenging passages in your life.

As I write, I envision us sitting down over a cup of coffee in my office or your kitchen as we work our way through many of the issues that you will be facing in the next few months. There is probably a box of tissues on the table, as well as pictures of your parents hanging on the wall.

Since I see this as a conversation, I use the "you and me" approach. I don't know if we are talking about your mother, father, in-laws, aunts, uncles, husband, or wife as we speak, so I have taken the liberty of alternating "mom" and "dad" for the person you are caring for. I have tried to stuff as much information as possible in these pages, but I know that this is only the starting point. In the appendix, you will find a list of resources for more in-depth information on payment systems, disease specific issues, and the like. I would strongly suggest you follow up with these as you have time.

To those families, residents, and clients I have worked with over the years, all of my examples are composites of real situations without any identifying information. Thank you for sharing your lives with me. I also want to salute all of those folks who work in senior care. You are my heroes. I thank you for all the things you do every single day of the year to make someone's life more comfortable and more meaningful.

A wonderful example of these dedicated people is my business partner and dear friend, Pam Hyder. Pam's first thought is always of how to make things better for our clients. Thanks Pam, for your humor and support in the writing of this book.

I dedicate this book to my parents, Bob and Troyetta Batley, who taught me the importance of a caring family, and to all of the families who care for loved ones each day.

Finally, I would like to express my profound appreciation to Steve Everhart and *The Senior's Choice*® for making this book possible. Steve's insights into the heart of senior care both motivate and inspire every member of *The Senior's Choice*®. Thank you Steve for your leadership!

With smiles and hugs,
Judy Castleberry

"Grow old with me!
The best is yet to be,
The last of life, for which the first was made."

Robert Browning

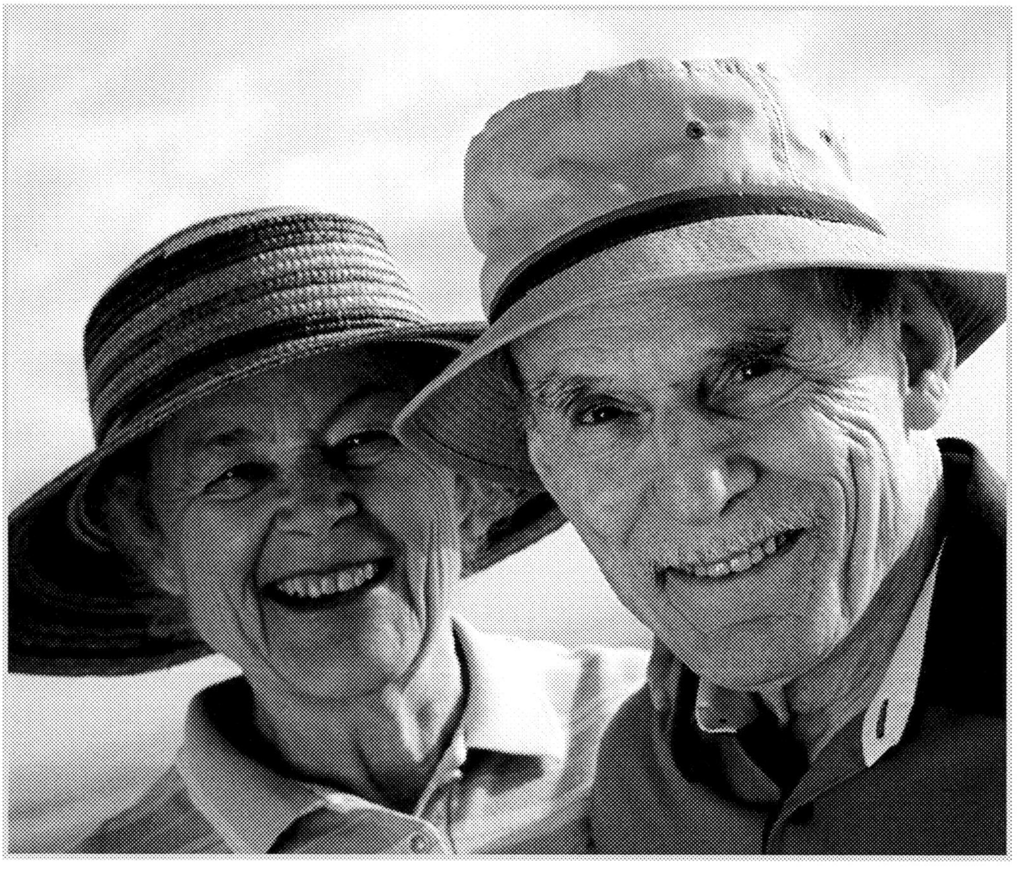

*"…they dropped off the work merry-go-round and retired.
We envied their carefree lifestyle…"*

CHAPTER ONE:

Your Ticket to The Zone

"Old age ain't for sissies."
Bette Davis

It's time to let out a dirty little secret: we are getting older. That means that if we are fortunate enough to still have them, our parents are too.

Of course, most of us think our parents have been old forever. After all, they were the old fogies who didn't approve of our music or the length of our hair or skirts back when we were teenagers. They got a lot smarter after we went to college and we let them in on all the neat stuff we learned. There was even a time when it seemed like we were catching up with them. After all, we were also worrying about jobs, bills, kids and marriages.

A few years ago, though, they dropped off the work merry-go-round and retired. We envied their carefree lifestyles tooling around the country in oversized RVs, playing golf or fishing. Some of them got involved in volunteer work and shamed us with their endless energy for SCORE, RSVP, and other senior volunteer groups.

However, if you picked up this book today, it is probably because you are about to enter another relationship with your parents. Something happened that made you realize you are about to enter "The Caregiver Zone."

BAD NEWS TRAVELS FAST

Ask any parent what is the worst phone call of their life and they will probably answer with some variation of:

"This is the police and we have your son . . . "

"This is the emergency room and we have your daughter."

We never think that someday we might receive another phone call that can be equally frightening. What do you do when the phone call is not about your teenager but about your elderly parent?

For me, the phone call came just as I was going into a daily staff meeting:

"Hi, I'm your mother's friend and she has had a bad fall. I am taking her to Immediate Care. Could you meet us there?"

As a long term care administrator, I have taken care of lots of other people's mothers. However, this was different. This was MY mother. My caregiver switch flipped on as I hurried across town to Immediate Care. Fortunately, my mother had only broken her wrist. Unfortunately, it was a very bad break and my father could not be reached by phone.

My parents (both in their early seventies) had been staying in their RV near a large lake about 50 miles from town. My father was fishing on his boat in the middle of this lake without any means of communication. My mother, in her continuing pursuit of cleanliness, had climbed up on the picnic table by their RV to knock down a nest that an enterprising sparrow had built under the edge of the metal shelter over the table. After succeeding in her mission, my mother lost her balance as she was climbing down. Momma's whole weight landed on her left wrist causing it to shatter.

That morning at the Immediate Care Center with my mother in intense pain and my father incommunicado, I had one of those "a-ha" moments: my parents are getting older. Apparently, the doctor thought so, too, because he carefully explained the fracture to me rather than my mother, the usual family caregiver. Whether it was her white hair or her pain, the medical people had cast me in the role of my mother's caregiver.

JUST A LITTLE HITCH IN MY GET-ALONG

Maybe you didn't get one of those calls. Maybe you just stopped by to visit your dad one day and noticed that his house smelled like the garbage hasn't been emptied in a long time. In his kitchen, the only food you find is cereal and chocolate chip cookies. Your dad, who was once named "Best Dressed" in his high school annual, is wearing clothes that have obviously not seen a washing machine in a long time.

Maybe your mom just gradually finds it too difficult to go to church and her club meetings. She complains about those crazy kids driving too fast—and she isn't talking about your boyfriend in his souped-up Chevy. Her car doesn't get moved very often and then one day it stops going all together. When you offer to get it fixed, she tells you not to bother.

Or, another variation of the phone calls happens. You live across the country and mom's neighbor calls:

"I'm your mother's next door neighbor. I really think you need to do something. I saw her in the front yard yesterday, naked as a jaybird."

That is when you know that nagging little doubt you have had in your mind suddenly becomes real. Your parents need help and you are elected caregiver. So now what do you do?

WHAT WOULD MOMMA DO?

There is a comfortable myth that in the "good old days" families just took care of their elderly. Remember the grandparents on "The Waltons"? Grandpa helped out at the lumber mill until he died and Grandma just kept on washing those dishes. If someone got sick, the doctor dropped by the house with his little black bag and mother boiled water or made chicken soup. Some of us remember multi-generational families living together. So why can't we take care of our elderly parents like they used to?

Answer Number One: The Numbers Game

In the good old days (think pre-1960) people just did not live as long. There were fewer old people to care for both in total number and as a percentage of the population. This was constant through the first half of the twentieth century. If grandma was over sixty-five, 94%-96% of the population was younger than she. If she was over eighty-five, almost everyone was younger than she. In real numbers, while there were only 122,000 Americans over the age of eighty-five in 1900, today there are close to 4.5 *million* and growing.

At the same time, the birthrate has gone down and we have become much more mobile with families stretched across the country. In the good old days, there were a lot more children and grandchildren to share the caregiving responsibilities for grandparents. Remember that while mom was making that chicken soup, her daughters were washing the dishes and the sons were fetching the wood for the stove.

In addition, since life expectancy was significantly shorter, grandmother did not need care for as long. After all, pneumonia was called the old man's friend for a reason. Today, antibiotics, aggressive surgeries, and other forms of treatment mean that illnesses or injuries that were life threatening only fifty years ago are now routinely treated and cured.

The longer life expectancy also introduces another difference between now and the world of "The Waltons": the "young old" are the caregivers for the "old old." It is very possible that you are in your sixties and taking care of a parent in his or her eighties. While you probably look and feel younger at sixty than your mother did, you are probably also still working to pay for your own retirement. You might even have a few twinges of arthritis yourself.

Answer Number Two: The Sicker/Healthier Conundrum

The reasons that people live longer—improved medical care, better food, less exposure to industrial accidents—also means that older people are healthier for a longer time. However, they are much sicker when they finally need care. According to the Centers for Disease Control (CDC), this change is evident when you compare nursing home admissions between 1985 and 1997. The folks admitted in 1997 needed more assistance and have a higher level of disability at admission.

The very medications, surgeries, and treatments that prolong life also produce more complicated long term care needs. When mom was taking care of grandmother, not only did she probably have a few siblings or children to help share the load, but grandmother was probably not as sick.

Yes, arthritis and old age have been around forever. But, when grandmother was cared for at home she probably did not have appointments with three doctors, insulin injections twice daily, sterile dressing changes, and seven medications that needed to be taken and monitored for reactions and side effects.

Today, treatment continues for conditions that might have been left untreated a few years ago, especially in the elderly. This means that you, as the family caregiver, need at least a basic understanding of how the medical system works because you will be dealing with a vast array of specialists, therapists, nurses, and other health care professionals. Even with the best intentions, these folks are usually too busy to really explain all of the ins and outs of arranging care.

Answer Number Three: The "Working Woman Thing"

While both men and women can be caregivers, in the past informal family caregiving was primarily the responsibility of the women of the family. Even if you would like to return to the old world where women only worked inside the home, the truth of the matter is that the vast majority of baby boomer women are also employed outside the home. If you are a man or a woman stepping into the Caregiver Zone, there is a more than fifty-fifty chance that you are employed full time. So are the rest of that informal network of adult daughters, daughters-in-law, neighbors, and friends who were available in years past to help out when Aunt Suzie had a spell of pneumonia.

In fact, one of the new realities you may be facing is the added struggle of maintaining a job while also being a caregiver. If you were in that first wave of working moms, you probably have some idea of what that means as you recall struggling to find good daycare for little Timmy, being passed over for promotions because you were considered less dependable, or fitting your work schedule around his school and activities. Unfortunately, your boss and co-workers are probably just a little clueless about how caregiving for an elderly parent may impact your work life. On the other hand, your boss may be all too aware as you are suddenly using up your sick leave taking care of dad.

In 1999, one of the first studies to look at this issue in depth was sponsored by MetLife Mature Market Institute and produced by the National Alliance for Caregiving, and the National Center on Women and Aging at Brandeis University. This study found that caregiving responsibilities impacted the caregiver in the workplace in such ways as reduced work hours, passing up job promotions or transfers, not being available to go for further training to enhance job skills, and other compromises that affected the caregiver financially and emotionally. It also affected the employer through lost productivity, absenteeism, and "presenteeism" where a person is present at work but not able to be productive due to exhaustion and stress.

By the way, even though the majority of the caregiving population is female, the reality is that many men are also struggling with the same issues. In fact, fully 25% of the households in our country are providing care for an elderly or handicapped individual. That's an awful lot of caregiving going on!

ENTERING THE CAREGIVER ZONE

So where are you in your journey through the Caregiver Zone? Did you just receive one of those phone calls? Are you just starting to notice some changes and are thinking ahead? Are you getting ready for your journey into the Caregiver Zone?

FIRST STEPS

By reading this book, you have taken a very important first step into the Caregiver Zone by gathering information. As we journey together through the Zone, we will look first at the emotional impact of becoming a caregiver. We will also look for signs of what kinds of intervention may be necessary, and when. The next part of our journey focuses on things to do before the "a-ha" moment—including finances and an overview of care options. The balance of the book is the nuts and bolts of caregiving in different situations. We end where we began by looking at your role as the family caregiver. By the way, if you are one of those folks who like to read the last chapter first, this is fine too. Sometimes you can't focus on caring for your folks until some of your needs are met. So if you are really hitting the end of your rope, now might be the right time to read that last chapter.

In addition, the appendix includes an example of an assessment for care, a glossary of common terms, and resources that will be very helpful as you travel through the Caregiver Zone.

THE REST OF THE STORY

Oh, by the way, my mother recovered fully from her shattered wrist. She never needed long term care. Despite two surgeries, she also never spent a night in a hospital. Medical care has changed dramatically since my mother went to nurse's training in the 1940's. A few years ago, this type of injury could have crippled her for life. Instead, she had a long uncomfortable summer with bi-weekly trips to an outpatient therapy clinic. Now she is back doing all of her normal activities. However, she's not standing on picnic tables!

At least for now, my "a-ha" moment was just that: only momentary. As a professional in senior care, I know that this could change again with another fall. Becoming a caregiver for your parents is truly one of the hardest challenges you will face in your life. However, you can get through it if you do your research, establish your team of helpers, and work with the professionals.

Welcome to the Caregiver Zone!

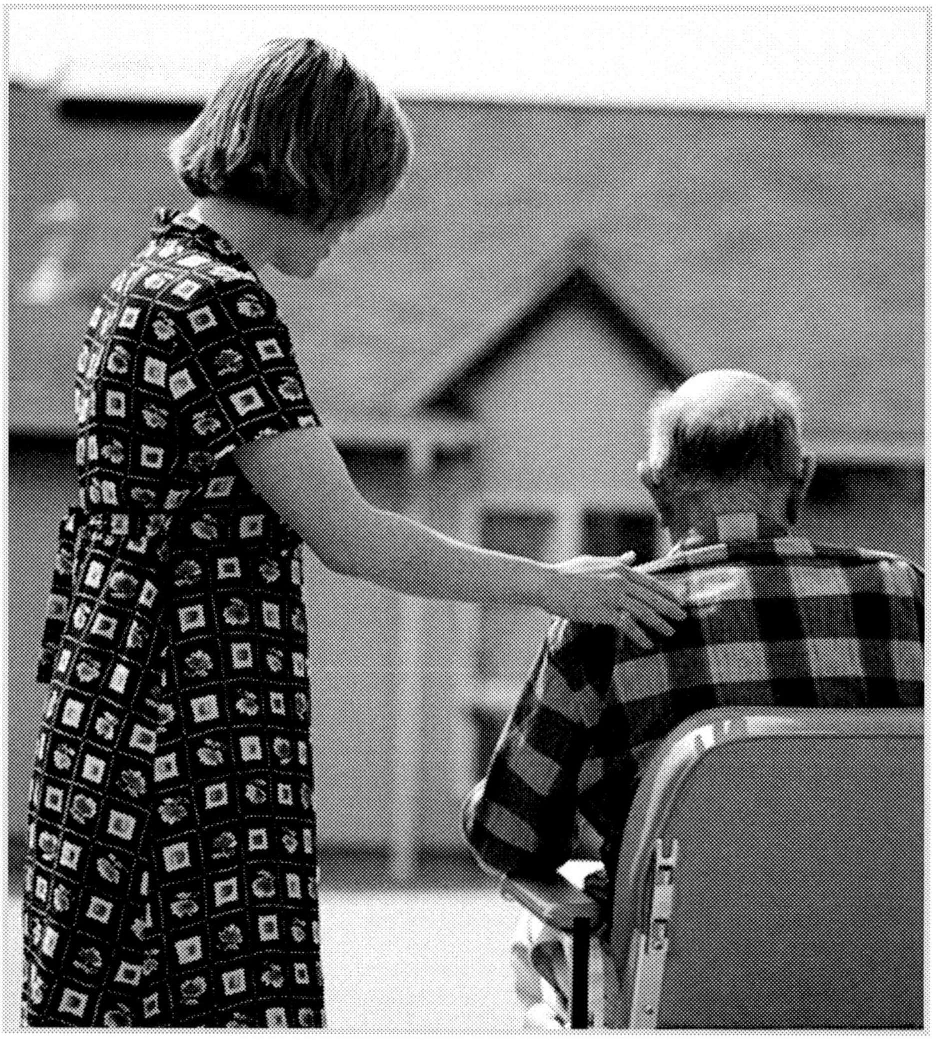

"…the next few days, weeks, or months will be the time for some major shifts in your relationship with your parent…"

CHAPTER TWO:

Tag, You're It!

"I ain't what I used to be, but who the hell is?"
Dizzy Dean

Along with all of the other roles in your life—employee, boss, wife, husband, mom, dad—you have suddenly added a new one: caregiver. So, what comes next? Do you feel like you need a medical degree or at least a master's degree in Medicare? What's the first thing to do?

Before you rush headlong into the caregiver maze, it might help to take a few minutes to look at what being a caregiver really means. It's not all about medication times and government programs. In fact, a lot of it is about how you (and your parents) deal with changes in your lives.

As a new caregiver, you will find that the next few days, weeks, or months will be the time for some major shifts in your relationship with your parent. While you are going through these shifts, don't forget the other side of the coin. Your parent is dealing with the double whammy of both the physical and/or mental changes that have caused them to need care and the reactions of folks around them, including you.

Remember when your children hit puberty? When you hit it yourself? Remember how no one seemed to really understand what a mess your life was?

Sometimes, that is how it feels to be an older person needing care. Your body doesn't seem to fit quite like it once did. The people around you are always saying stupid things like "act your age" or "you are too old/young to understand." It isn't that your parents have suddenly become teenagers. After all, they have a lifetime of skills and memories to draw upon. It is just that nothing looks or feels quite right, like a reflection in a fun house mirror. Scary, isn't it?

So, before we get really confused, let's look at a few reactions to the "a-ha" moment that tend to create more problems than they solve.

FIVE THINGS NOT TO DO AT THE "A-HA" MOMENT

1. THE "DO-SOMETHING" SYNDROME

When mankind faced saber-tooth tigers on a regular basis, we needed the rush of adrenaline to give us the strength and speed to run for our lives. This reaction saved enough of our ancestors that we are here now today. Unfortunately, what is often the best thing to do when facing saber-tooth tigers can be the worst thing to do when confronting issues with aging parents.

For many folks the first reaction to the "a-ha" moment is that they must do something—and the faster the better. For example, Sally comes home for a visit and realizes that her mother has not been eating right for a long time. Sally insists that her mother immediately move across country to live with her so she can take care of mom. Sally doesn't think about the home that mom has lived in for forty years or her friends at church. Surely, mom can just make new friends at her new church when she gets to feeling better. At Sally's home, mom continues to eat poorly and refuses to go to the new church with Sally. Instead, she sits staring out the window all day fretting about what is happening to her yard back home.

The "Do Something" Syndrome also appears in medical situations. People often expect medicine to operate at the breakneck speed of an ER episode: all sirens, flashing lights, and shocking people back to life. The reality is that most medical care, especially geriatric care, moves at a slower pace.

"Why isn't the doctor doing something?" or "I'm going to take my mother to ____ (whatever the closest big city is) to a better doctor" or "I want my mother on the magic pill I saw advertised on TV the other night." While all of these might be good responses, the reality is they also might not be. This panicky demand that something, *anything*, be done immediately can really get in the way of finding a good solution to your mother's care.

On the other hand, if it doesn't seem that the medical people are paying attention to all of mom's symptoms, don't be afraid to speak up. If you are the primary caregiver, you will probably see symptoms before anyone else does. Don't feel that just because you don't have letters after your name you are incapable of seeing changes in health and behavior.

2. PRETEND IT WILL GO AWAY

This is a good solution for ostriches, but it does not work very well for caregivers. This is an especially easy game to play if you live at a distance. After all, dad still sounds the same on the phone. He is still talking about football and cars. Surely, everything is all right.

While doing in-home assessments for companion care, I usually check the bathroom for safety devices. In more homes than you would expect, the bathtub or shower has obviously not been used in a long time. Clothes are hung on the shower curtain rod, there is no soap or shampoo nearby, or a heavy chair or other item is sitting in the way. The adult children who assure me that mom or dad shower daily are usually surprised when I point this out. One of the surprising discoveries about the Caregiver Zone is how often we overlook the obvious. Keep your eyes and ears open for clues about care needs.

3. THE BLAME GAME

There are two parts to this game. The first is blaming the victim. Anyone who has smoked cigarettes in the last twenty years and is not comatose knows that smoking is harmful. The same can also be said for overuse of alcohol, food, prescription and non-prescription drugs. Because we have this information, some folks have got it figured out that if everyone just does healthy things no one would ever get sick.

While I am not advocating smoking four packs of cigarettes a day or living on a diet of Twinkies, the reality is that people can live a totally healthy lifestyle and still get sick. Moreover, even if bad habits contributed to the current illness, this is probably not the time to try to change someone's entire lifestyle. They probably won't change and will only resent you for trying to make them.

The second part of the blame game is to blame someone else, often a sibling: blame the brother who lives out of area for not visiting more often, blame the sister who lives a block away for not watching out better for the folks, blame the youngest for worrying mom, blame the oldest for not taking the keys away. After a while it all starts sounding pretty ridiculous, but this is often how families deal with crisis. Don't waste your energy on the blame game. Save it for the more important task of caring for your parent.

4. GUILT TRIPS

The flip side of the blame game is the "It's all my fault" game. If only I hadn't moved to Chicago, if only I had noticed dad's Alzheimer's earlier, if only I hadn't lied about skipping school in eighth grade. Okay, that last one is a little farfetched, but some of the other guilt trips I have seen people give themselves are almost as strange.

Just like you are not going to stop your father from smoking after thirty-nine years, you cannot go back and change the past. In reality, a lot of what you are blaming yourself for probably is not what made the difference. Even if you had not moved to Chicago your mother would still have had a stroke. The reason you did not notice your dad's Alzheimer's is he covered it so well. As far as the childhood secrets, give yourself a break. Forgiving yourself for the past is part of putting it behind you. You are going to need it behind you because you have a lot to take care of in front of you.

5. I'M IN CHARGE NOW!

I met a woman who became a caregiver for both of her parents while still in her twenties. When asked how she had managed, her reply was, "Well I just sat them down and told them how it was going to be, that I was in charge now." While I don't know how her parent's responded, I do know what my reaction would be if my twenty-something child said this to me!

Very few people respond calmly when the kid that they taught how to walk is now telling them how to do it. When you are appointed caregiver, trying to remember that your parents are still in charge is sometimes the greatest challenge of all. I can already hear someone saying, *"But my mother has dementia. That means I must make the decisions, right?"* Right, but wrong.

Not all decisions are life and death. Why take away someone's decisions about foods, lifestyles, where they live, etc? Even as a parent travels down the road to dementia, try to give them every opportunity to stay in charge of their life. It will make their life, as well as yours, better.

It is extremely important to remember that even in a dementia situation, this is not your life. This is your mom or dad's life. Understanding *their* values is the bottom line when making decisions. While it may seem more cumbersome, being guided by your parent's wishes will make most decisions become easier in the long run. The next chapter outlines some tools to help you understand your parent's values.

WHEN THE CAREGIVER IS THE SPOUSE

So far in this book, we have mainly talked about the caregiver as an adult child. However, in our country 62% of caregivers are spouses. There are special challenges for the caregiver spouse. Suddenly those wedding vows of "for better or worse, in sickness and in health" have new meaning. If your spouse needs care, there is a good possibility that you are also getting up in years. Maybe you have health problems of your own that preclude you providing physical care for your husband or wife. You may even still be working or raising children or grandchildren.

Years ago, a wife of one of my nursing home residents told me, "Sometimes I think it would be easier if I were a widow. My friends just don't understand what it is like when I don't know if he even realizes I come to visit him." As hard as it is to deal with the death of a spouse, at least there are accustomed roles to fill. Friends and family rally around you and strangers try to help. However, when your spouse is sick, your role as caregiver is often the hardest. Later, we will look at coping as the caregiver spouse. In the meantime, remember that the term caregiver in this book includes YOU.

WHEN DOING SOMETHING IS THE RIGHT ANSWER

Now that we have run through the DON'T list, it's time to look at the DO list. The next chapters are full of information regarding issues for caregivers. But how do you decide that it is time to do anything at all?

When I started working in nursing homes in 1980, the prevailing wisdom was that we restrained people in wheelchairs to keep them safe. The idea was if someone was tied in a chair they would not fall. So caring professionals and families worked together to tie fragile old people into wheelchairs for their own safety.

A few years later, several studies were done that proved that restraints actually caused falls as well as dehydration, poor circulation, and overall decline. By trying to protect people from falling, we were actually making them less safe.

You might not be considering restraints, but sometimes the same thought process is in the works. Which is riskier: moving your fragile parent or caring for him/her in place? Moving across the country, admission to a facility, even intervention in the home are all big steps that may have unforeseen consequences. How do you weigh these risks?

The answer comes in the concept of "acceptable risk." Every day we each make decisions on what risks we are willing to take. Which is riskier: driving through traffic to work or staying home? If not going to work means that you could lose your job, which in turn would cause great harm to your family, this might not be an acceptable risk. On the other hand, choosing between routes through a lot of freeway construction versus a safer route that avoids the construction might be an acceptable risk.

As you look at intervening in your parents' lives, ask yourself the following questions while keeping in mind the idea of acceptable risk. What risks are acceptable to your parents? What risks are acceptable to you? It might be a good idea to return to these questions on those days when every decision seems to lead to more confusion.

WHEN SHOULD I WORRY?

- Would I be afraid for my parent if I left town for a weekend? A week? A month?
- Has there been a significant change in health status such as a large weight gain or loss, recent hospitalization, new medication regime, etc.?
- Would my parent be able to summon help if they had a medical or other emergency?
- Is my parent's home safe? Can unsafe conditions in the home be made safer with grab bars, more lighting, or a little fix up?
- Which is most important to my parent--safety or independence? If safety and independence are on opposite ends of the scale, where is my parent right now?
- Am I worrying about medical concerns or lifestyle choices? What harm will come about if they continue in their lifestyle choice?
- What is the least that can be done to produce the best result?

The last question in this chart refers to the medical principal of providing care in the least restrictive environment. In later chapters, we will be talking about the vast array of services available for elderly parents. While services can be provided in a number of settings, most people are happiest in the setting where they feel there are the fewest restraints on their independence.

By the way, if you weren't able to answer all of the questions above, don't be discouraged about your progress through this maze. Just knowing what the questions are is the first step toward getting the answers. The next chapter will give you some tools for finding the answers that keep your parents in charge of their lives while keeping some sanity in yours.

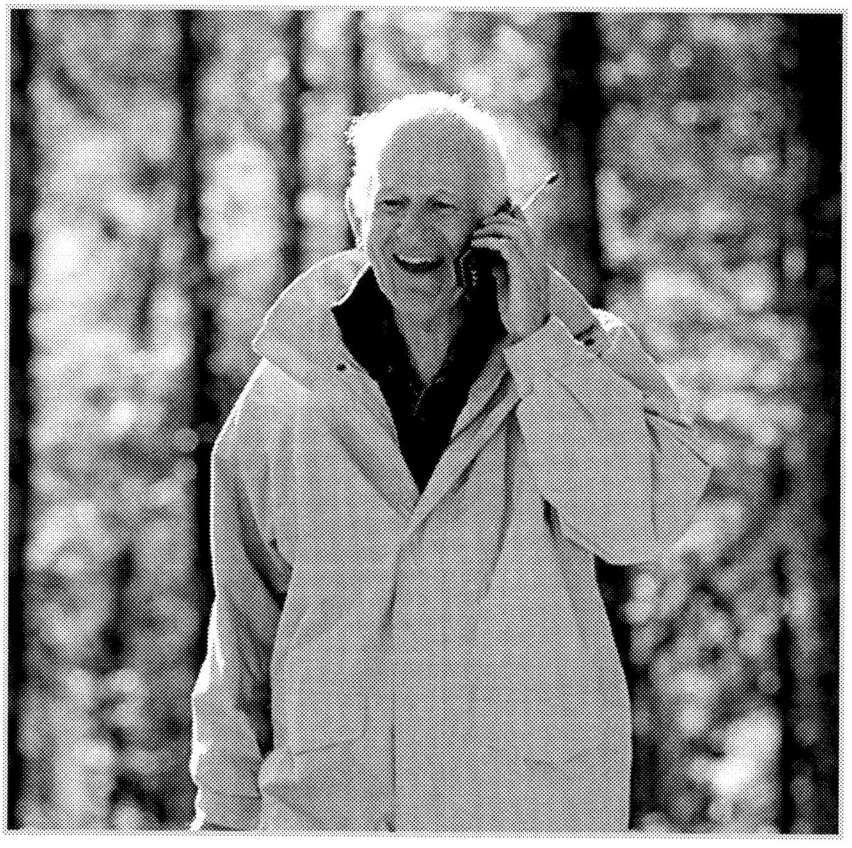

"...for safety reasons, all of us, whether we are 17, 47, or 87 need to share certain information about ourselves with other people..."

CHAPTER THREE:

Being Prepared Isn't Just for Boy Scouts

"Can you hear me now?"
Verizon Commercial

START TALKING

In the twenty-plus years I have been involved in senior care, I have known thousands of families including a few that probably belonged on "The Jerry Springer Show." However, most families are really trying to make things better for their parents. Unfortunately, good intentions don't always have good results. What seems to make the difference is the ability to understand and respect the values of the parents, even when you don't agree with them.

We are the generation with every possible device for instant communication all over the globe. However, when it comes to understanding our own parents, the cell phones, email, and instant messaging alone just don't seem to work. Opening the lines of communication with your parents is probably the most important step to help you and your parents through the caregiver maze.

Every family has developed a pattern of communication or non-communication. For example, my family operates by committee. I am the middle of five sisters and family meetings to discuss holiday plans or care for a sick family member are the norm. My family tends to be verbal and this works for us.

You need to figure out what works for your family. Or, at least develop a truce so that the real issues involved in care can be discussed. While you might not be able to solve the old bitter family history, opening the channels of communication between parent and child as well as between siblings will help everyone, especially the caregiver and care receiver. Later, we will talk more about getting help from your siblings if you are the primary caregiver.

So, what do you need to communicate about? In the next few months and years, you may be put in a position where you will be asked to make decisions regarding care. While some things (deciding to go to the doctor for a check-up) are fairly simple, other decisions (how far to take treatment for cancer) might not be as simple. This is where understanding your mom or dad's values will make the difference.

Talking openly about these types of issues does not come naturally in many families. Even if you and your siblings visit mom and dad regularly, it is often easier to discuss the weather or the outcome of the Sunday afternoon game. Whatever the excuse, these are some hints to help get the conversation going:

- Set a time for a family discussion. A quick phone call from across the country or dropping by during your dad's favorite TV show might not be the best time for this type of discussion.
- If you have siblings, include them in the discussion. Just remember the focus is to remain on your parents' values and needs, not on old issues between siblings.
- Assure your parents that you just want to make sure you understand their wishes should there ever be a need for you to help with decisions.
- Use a guide such as a Values History Form to help open up the conversation and keep it on task.
- Listen to what is said. You are there to receive information, not argue, bring up the missed tenth birthday, or pass judgment.
- Listen to what isn't said. Sometimes parents don't want to bring up an issue because they are afraid it might upset you. Watch for cues that something more needs to be said.
- Realize that for many older people the most important thing is just to be heard. We all want to feel that we are in control of our own lives.

- Understand that not everything has an immediate answer or maybe any answer at all. That's all right. Life doesn't usually come in neat packages.

FIRST THINGS FIRST

Now that you have the family gathered around the kitchen table, what are you going to talk about? The box below contains sample questions that can be a good beginning to a family discussion. Remember, there are no right or wrong answers, just opinions. After living with your parents for at least eighteen years, you might think you know their values. Most people change somewhat as they age. What was important to your parents when they had a house full of teenagers or were planning their retirement might no longer be as important. So listen up and learn what interesting folks your parents really are.

SAMPLE VALUES QUESTIONS

1. How would you describe your current health status? If you currently have any medical problems, how would you describe them?
2. How difficult is it for you to maintain the kind of environment for yourself that you find comfortable? Does any illness or medical problem you have now mean that it will be harder in the future?
3. Do you think you would want to have any of the following medical treatments performed on you: kidney dialysis, CPR, respirator, artificial nutrition, artificial hydration, or other suggested treatments?
4. How important is independence and self-sufficiency in your life? If you were to experience decreased physical and mental abilities, how would that affect your attitude toward independence and self-sufficiency?

5. If you would no longer be able to make decisions regarding your health and medical care, who would you want to make these decisions? Have you made any legal arrangements for this?
6. What would you fear most about a terminal illness?
7. What, if any, unfinished business from the past are you concerned about (e.g., personal and family relationships, business and legal matters)?
8. What goals do you have for the future?
9. How much do you worry about having enough money to provide for your care?
10. What role do your religious beliefs play in your life? How do your religious beliefs affect your attitude toward serious or terminal illness?
11. What is your greatest joy in life?

Excerpt from Values History form developed at the Institute of Public Law, University of New Mexico, through a grant from the Ittleson Foundation. The complete form can be found at lawschool.unm.edu/Clinic/resources/healthcare/index.htm.

GETTING IT ON PAPER

With the right approach, you may have a few more insights into how your parents think. If that is all you gain from this kind of discussion, then it has been well worth the time. However, it might be a good idea to go to the next step: getting it on paper.

In the old west, a man's handshake was his bond. Many years the crops or cattle were sent to market based on a verbal agreement that the buyer would pay the seller a fair price. Unfortunately, in our litigious society, we can no longer rely on handshakes. Instead, the written word, properly executed is needed. The next stop in the maze is the alley of legal documents. This is an important place to journey through BEFORE there is a problem.

WHAT IS ALL THAT PAPER FOR ANYWAY?

- **Advance Directive** is sometimes used as an umbrella term for any document that directs healthcare or care for the terminal patient. It can also mean a separate document that spells out in detail such decisions as whether or not to intubate, recessitate, or perform other medical procedures.

- **A Living Will** tells your doctor to withdraw life-sustaining treatment if two doctors agree that you are no longer able to make decisions and you are terminally ill, irreversibly unconscious, or in a permanent vegetative state. Think in terms of life threatening accidents, comas, or end-stage illnesses.

- **Durable Healthcare Power of Attorney** is more general than a living will. It says that your parent is assigning someone else, such as a spouse or adult child, to make healthcare decisions when they can't due to loss of mental ability or advance illness.

- **Durable Power of Attorney** is used to appoint someone else to make decisions regarding your finances. By the way, a power of attorney that does not say it is durable, or stays in effect when the person is incompetent, is invalid once this happens. Many old standard powers of attorney did not include this and so the very fact that mom now can't make decisions makes the old power of attorney useless.

- **A Will** provides the individual's directions regarding how property is to be distributed, and appoints a person (the executor) to make sure that the individual's wishes are carried out.

DO I NEED A LAWYER?

Just as do-it-yourself surgery is not usually considered a good idea, neither is being a do-it-yourself lawyer. Water cooler talk about your co-worker's brother-in-law's mother does not necessarily apply to your mother. State laws, marital status, competency, prior legal documents, and other circumstances can have a profound effect on any of the documents listed above.

Lawyers have become specialists, just like doctors. Elder law is one of these specialties. The real estate attorney who did a great job when you bought your house might not be the right person to assist with the complexities of your parent's will or advance directives. The best free legal advice you will ever hear is to find an attorney with expertise in elder law. The Resource Listing gives you some national places to start searching for the right lawyer for you and your family, including some free services.

WHEN YOU SEE THE LAWYER

As you are wandering into the legal alleyway, there are a few additional issues to consider. One of the most important is the question of WHEN to develop advance directives. The answer is BEFORE there are any problems with dad's mental status. This is because legal documents must be signed while the individual signing the document is still competent to understand and make rational decisions. It is not legal to have your mother, who can no longer remember the names of her grandchildren (or even that she has them), to sign documents to preserve assets for those grandchildren. In fact, if your attorney indicates that it is still okay for mom to sign a new advance directive at this point, run—don't walk—away from him as fast as you can. This is not legal or ethical.

Another issue to consider when choosing a lawyer is that laws differ in each state. The Karen Ann Quinlin case in Missouri would not have happened in some states because of differences in the statutes regarding the right to die. It is important that your lawyer be familiar with the laws in the state where your parents reside. If you live in California and your parents live in Massachusetts, they need a

Massachusetts lawyer.

By the way, hospitals, nursing homes, or other healthcare providers are required to ask if the patient has any advance directives. This is not to be intrusive or to imply that they will be needed soon, but to make sure that the healthcare provider is aware of the wishes of the patient. In addition, it is not required that anyone have these documents in order to be admitted.

Since these documents are not required, what happens if your dad does not have them? Again, this depends on state law. In most states, there is an order of precedence regarding who gets to make decisions when no one is designated. It might run something like this: spouse, parents, adult children, adult siblings, other family members, interested parties. In some situations, this might be fine. However, what if your parents are estranged or your siblings disagree with each other or with your father regarding the care of your mother? Do you really want an "interested party" making life and death decisions for you?

By the way, while you are encouraging your parents to talk to a lawyer about these, make an appointment for yourself. Anyone could be in an automobile accident tomorrow.

YOU GOTTA HAVE FILES

Now that you have these documents, what do you do with them? And what about the rest of the paperwork that suddenly seems so important?

The following lists are documents that you should have organized by a suggested place to file them. Make duplicates as needed so the right person has the document at the right time. It really does not do a lot of good to have the only copy of a living will locked up in an attorney's office or a safe deposit box. Emergencies always happen at the most inconvenient time, such as long holiday weekends when banks and offices are closed.

Your Parent's Purse or Wallet

- Driver's license

- Insurance Card(s)
- Medicare, VA, and/or Medicaid Card
- Medical Alert Information or major diagnosis
- Current list of medications
- Emergency phone numbers such as the doctor or family members

Hint: Every few months, check that the information is current. Photocopy everything on the list and keep the copy where it is readily accessible to you. You will appreciate having done this when you are standing in the emergency room.

Magnets on Your Parent's Refrigerator

- Medical Alert Information or major diagnosis
- Current list of medications
- List of emergency phone numbers
- Location of advance directives in house

Hint: Some ambulance companies train their folks to look on the refrigerator for this kind of information.

Filed Where You Can Easily Find Them

- Copies of all Advance Directives
- List of numbers:

Social Security	*Medicare*
Medicaid	*VA*

Health Insurance *Life Insurance*

Bank Accounts/Safety Deposit Box

- In Case of Death Information

  Burial Plots

  Pre-need contracts

  Life Insurance Policies

  Pension Information

  Final Wishes

Hint: If you have any concerns about your mom or dad's mental competency, make copies and keep at your house for safekeeping. Folks have been known to put papers away for safekeeping and they are never found again.

Other Information

In the next chapter, we will be discussing financial resources at greater length, but while you are organizing documents keep in mind that certain programs such as Medicaid, Veterans Administration, or HUD will have lists of documents required to prove eligibility. A few of these documents are:

- Bank Statements
- Pay Stubs
- Birth Certificate or proof of citizenship
- Military discharge papers
- Life Insurance Policies
- Divorce Decrees

- Any other financial records such as loan papers, property deeds, proof of sale of assets, etc.

If you will be helping your parent qualify for this type of program, ask for a copy of any application or other form that you complete for the program. Keep it with all of your supporting documents.

This is also a good time to invest in a file box to keep medical billing information. Each time your parent is seen by the doctor or any other medical provider several documents will be generated: the original checkout bill, the Medicare Explanation of Benefits (EOB), and possibly an insurance Explanation of Benefits. These should be kept together in case there is a billing error and for tax records.

FINAL THOUGHT

As you become more intimately involved in your mom's business, look back again to your teenage years. One of the sure signs of puberty is when a child's bedroom door suddenly seems to be closed more often than open. That kid who once needed mom to lie beside him to lull him back to sleep after a nightmare, suddenly doesn't even want mom in his room. The amount of information that gets passed on to parents seems to drop to the "Yeah," "Out," and "I need money" level. Teenagers know instinctively that giving information is giving up control. However, good parents need to know where their kids are and what they are doing. Deep down, that kid who is shrugging his shoulders at you knows this too.

Adults also have the need for privacy, especially regarding issues as personal as medical and financial information. However, for safety reasons, all of us—whether we are seventeen, forty-seven, or eighty-seven—need to share certain information about ourselves with other people. If you were the one hit by the truck tomorrow, would your family be equipped to take care of the business side of your life?

Keep this in mind when handling information from your parents. Look at it as a backup system for when "something happens." The goal is to keep your folks in charge of their own life as much as possible at every stage. The whole purpose of this information gathering is to make sure your parents are cared for according to their values.

With all this information, are you starting to feel all dressed up withno place to go? Then take a deep breath, because the next bend in the maze is going to take us to the thicket of finances and government programs. This is where a lot of critical decisions will be made.

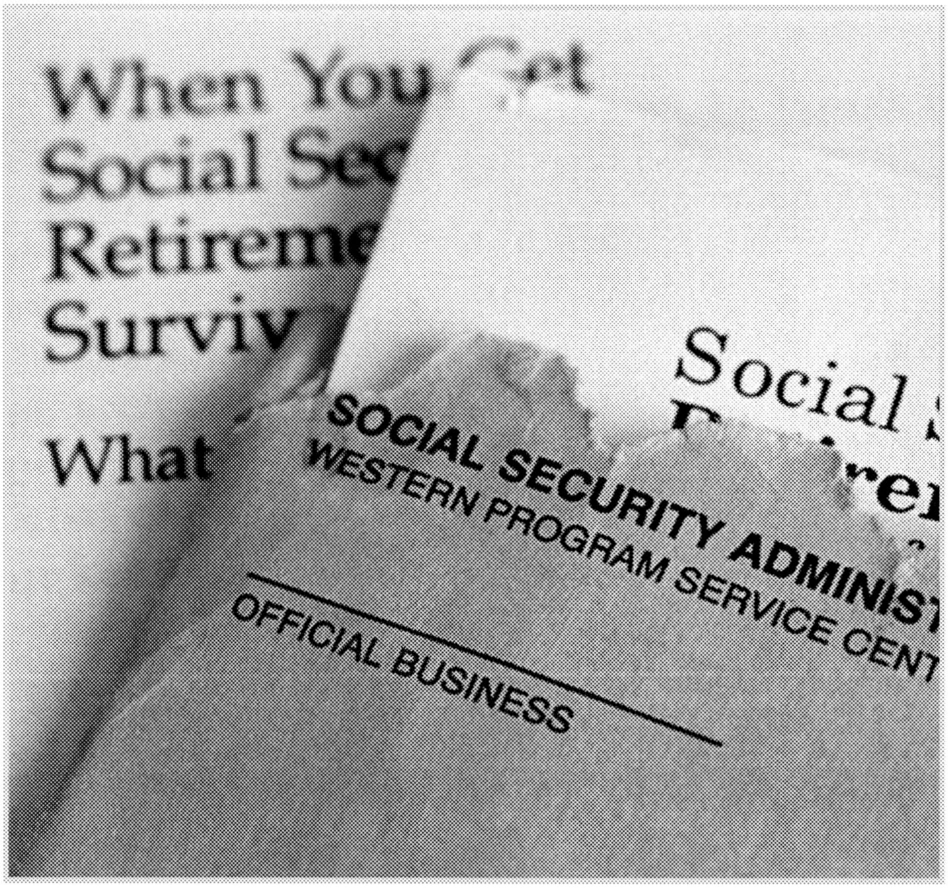

"…it is extremely important that you understand how payers influence the care your parents receive…"

CHAPTER FOUR:

Paying for It

"We're Spending Our Children's Inheritance"
Bumper Sticker seen on an RV

THE MAGIC WORLD OF MEDICARE AND MEDICAID

A long time ago (1938 to be exact), the wise rulers of a magic kingdom decided to help the old folks of their kingdom pay for medical care by creating a small insurance program. It was only for the old folks (over sixty-five) and only took care of major expenses like the hospital and the doctor. They dubbed this program "Medicare" as it was medical care for the elderly.

A few years later, the wise rulers of this kingdom also realized that many poor people, including children and old folks who needed more than Medicare paid for, could not afford to pay for medical care. Therefore, these wise and compassionate rulers created another program to pay for medical care for poor people. The rulers decided to attach the program to the many other programs that were being created in the fiefdoms that were a part of the kingdom. "Medicaid" was the name for this new program as it was medical financial aid.

In the years following these modest beginnings, new rulers added on to the programs to include more deserving people. They also added rules to make sure that no one who was not worthy received the benefits from these programs. Knights were added to watch over the healthcare providers who received payment from these programs. Thus, the simple little programs turned into the mysterious world of Medicare and Medicaid.

STICKER SHOCK

Isn't it nice that those wise rulers created Medicare and Medicaid? Now mom and dad are taken care of for life, right? WRONG! One of the first shocks you will probably have as you enter the Caregiver Zone is the reality of what things cost. And a tummy-churning second dose of reality hits when you discover how little of it is paid for by other folks.

Senior care is not cheap. Just as an example, the average daily cost of nursing home care in 2002 was over $150 per day, with a range from $448 in Alaska to $99 in Louisiana according to the AARP Public Policy Institute. These rates tend to rise 3%-6% per year. As I will explain in more detail later, Medicare pays for very little of this care. So, be prepared to ask lots of questions about price. That nest egg your folks put away for a rainy day is probably going to disappear rapidly in the next few months and years.

THE GOLDEN RULE: HE WHO HAS THE GOLD MAKES THE RULES

OK, maybe that sounds a little cynical. Unless you are independently wealthy and pay cash for all healthcare, it is extremely important that you understand how payers influence the care your parents receive. In healthcare, the payers set rules regarding how, where, and sometimes how much care will be provided. These payers include Medicare, Medicaid, Veterans Administration, other government payers, and insurance. Even if you or your parents pay for services directly, payers still control the services you will receive because over the years most providers have developed their programs around these payment sources.

Confused? Don't feel alone. One of the deep dark secrets of healthcare is that most providers are a little confused, too. That is because each of these payment systems (Medicare, Medicaid, insurances, etc.) has slightly different rules. A provider may be receiving payment for your mom's care from many sources, all of which have different payment rules. This is why it is so important for you to have at least a general grasp of how payment systems work.

The Catch-22 of Payers

The minute you think you understand the rules on payment for healthcare they will change. Sometimes they will change in ways that are advantageous to your parents; sometimes the changes will be disastrous to your parents. The only constant is that the payment system will change. If a provider or any other advisor gives you information about a payment system that seems conflicting or inaccurate, check with your payment source for accuracy. The final authority is the payment source.

When you are confronting the issues of who pays for what in healthcare there are three primary questions that need to be answered:

1. Is the person eligible for the payment source?
2. Is the service covered by the payment source?
3. Is the provider certified to receive payment from this payment source?

Frankly, since most providers are skilled at finding ways to pay for their services, if numbers one and two are taken care of, you can usually find number three fairly easily. Now we will look at the general rules to help you understand numbers one and two. The provider side will be covered more thoroughly in the next few chapters.

WE ARE FROM THE GOVERNMENT AND WE ARE HERE TO HELP

One of those funny things people like to say, but don't really think through is that they don't want "the government" messing in healthcare. The reality is that government is the largest payer of healthcare in our country. Veterans Administration, Public Health Service, Indian Health Service, and, of course, Medicare and Medicaid are all possible sources of payment for care for your parents. Since Medicare and Medicaid are the most prevalent—and most easily confused—we are going to talk about them in the most detail.

It is too bad that when those smart people in Washington first invented these programs they weren't a little more creative with the names. But since the names are so similar, here are a few of the differences:

IS IT MEDICARE OR MEDICAID?

	Medicare	Medicaid
Eligibility	Age, Disability, paid into system	Financial Need, Medically Eligible
Premiums	Part A - taxes Part B - monthly premium	No premiums
Who Runs It	Federal Program	State Program with federal oversight
Portability	National	Different program in each state
Covered services	Acute, skilled services	Lots of different programs including unskilled services
Application process	Automatic with Social Security, or simple application form	Extensive financial review process, certain programs also require medical eligibility
Age requirements	Sixty-five or certain disabilities	All ages including children of low income families

MEET MR. MEDICARE

At its heart, Medicare is a medical insurance system. As you can see by the chart, you become eligible by paying into the system through your Social Security taxes for Part A and by paying a premium for Part B. Like other insurances, it has an annual deductible and co-pays.

Part A is hospital insurance to take care of the major problems in life, including hospitalization and skilled services that continue after the hospital (examples are home health care agencies or skilled units in long term care facilities). These are sometimes also referred to as "inpatient services" or "skilled services." In other words, these procedures were historically done inpatient in a hospital by a skilled medical worker such as a doctor, nurse, or therapist. Hospice care also falls into this category.

Part B is medical insurance for services beyond the hospital such as doctor visits, out patient hospital care, durable medical equipment, and out patient therapies. In order to have this, your parents are paying a monthly premium.

By the way, the easiest way to find out if your parents have both parts is to look at their Medicare card. It will list "Part A" and "Part B."

The next issue in Medicare is where it gets complicated. A few years ago, when everyone thought that HMOs would be the saving grace of healthcare, seniors were given the option of using their Medicare benefit to purchase Medicare+Choice plans operated by private insurance companies. The insurance companies had to cover certain basic benefits under Medicare, but could choose to add benefits or contain costs by requiring the patient to use their network. Since these plans can differ from insurance company to insurance company, they tend to be more regionalized.

One of the good things about Medicare is that it is a federal program. Even though there are regional fiscal agents such as the various Blue Cross/Blue Shields, in general, the benefits that are paid for in Maine will be the same benefits paid in Arizona. In our mobile society, this is important when mom and dad hitch up the RV to move to Arizona for the winter. However, if your parent has a Medicare+Choice plan, check with the plan when moving your parent. If the move is a large distance, you might be surprised to find out that the plan is not always portable. The good news here is that you can opt out of the plan at any time and return to standard Medicare.

For more information about Medicare, check out the website at *medicare.gov*. Your parents should also receive a Medicare handbook each year that explains the current program.

MEDICAID, THE POOR RELATION

If your parents need financial help to pay for care at home or in a facility, you may need to apply for Medicaid. In most states this is done through a county or city income support office. If your parents have always paid their own way, this may be the first time they have ever had to apply for a government program. Be forewarned, a Medicaid application is usually a lengthy intrusive process. Make friends with your caseworker because you are going to need his/her help to get through this process.

Because Medicaid is state specific, it would be impossible to explain all of the programs available in each state through the Medicaid program. Instead, here are a few general issues to keep in mind while exploring the Medicaid branch of the Caregiver Zone.

- Medicaid is not just one program, but an umbrella for a wide range of financial aid programs. Each program has specific eligibility requirements. Your parents might qualify for some programs but not others.
- Eligibility and benefits vary from state to state. Just because someone qualifies in one state does not mean they automatically qualify in another, even a neighboring state. There are also residency requirements in most states so if your parent is moving, be sure to contact the Medicaid offices as early as possible so that you don't have a bad surprise during the move.
- Do not assume that your parents qualify or don't qualify for Medicaid based on general guidelines. Medicaid has a lot of exemptions and special rules that must be considered. The only way to really know if someone qualifies is to apply.
- This shouldn't have to be said, but it is important to be honest with the Medicaid office. Hiding assets is considered fraud and your parents can lose benefits, be sued, and/or have to pay back anything paid on their behalf by the Medicaid program. I've seen this happen and it is really ugly.
- Be wary of anyone who says that they can show you how to divert assets so that your parent will qualify for Medicaid while maintaining your inheritance. States can look back 36 months for transfers of assets. This means that your parents would need to have the foresight to transfer all of their assets to someone else more than 36 months before qualifying for Medicaid. Most people cannot predict three years ahead when they are going to need Medicaid.

OTHER GOVERNMENT PAYERS

Now that you have played with the big M's, don't forget that there are other payment sources within the government.

If your dad (and don't forget mom) is a veteran, it is worth checking into VA benefits. VA provides care directly at clinics, hospitals, and through long term care agencies. It also pays for care through other providers with VA contracts. VA pensions are also available. Even if dad already receives a VA pension, check with the VA to see if it could be improved. There are special programs for former POWs and others with service-connected disabilities. Like Medicaid, be prepared to have to wade through a lot of qualifying paperwork, but it can be very helpful once you are inside the system.

Like VA, Indian Health Services is both a provider and a payer of healthcare. Qualifying for IHS is usually through proof of Native American heritage. Contact the Tribal Health Office for further information.

INSURANCE AND OTHER STRANGERS

Insurance is the thing you buy hoping you will never need it. Whether you buy insurance independently or through an employer, union, or other group, the basic premise is that a lot of people pool their funds for a rainy day. Health insurance is for when someone gets pneumonia from all that rain.

There are several kinds of insurance that your folks may own that help cover the cost of care: health insurance, Medigap, long term care, or life insurance. This is another branch of the maze that many people find confusing, so let's sort it out.

Health Insurance

If your dad is too young to qualify for Medicare or does not qualify for other reasons, he may have health insurance through a private company. Usually standard health insurance covers doctor's visits, hospitalizations, home health agencies, and other standard treatment costs. The problem is that it does not usually cover long term care facilities, assisted living, or anything considered "non-medical." Talk to the insurance company to find out exactly what it will and won't cover.

Medigap

This is the insurance to fill in the gaps in Medicare, such as the deductibles and co-pays. This might not sound like much, but those co-pays can really add up fast. Just as an example, the total co-pay for the twenty-first through 100th day in a skilled facility is currently $8400. (Medicare pays the entire charge for the first twenty days.)

By the way, Medicaid will often give an allowance to keep your Medigap insurance in effect. They figure it is cheaper to pay the premium than take on all of your co-pays and deductibles.

Long Term Care Insurance

This is one of the new kids on the block. Long term care insurance is usually a policy you buy separately from other insurance. A few employee cafeteria programs are now offering it as an add-on to health insurance. The time to buy long term care insurance is when you are a healthy fifty year-old because the premiums increase rapidly with age. Most companies won't even sell your mom a policy if she is over eighty or has certain pre-existing conditions.

Think of long term care insurance as an alternative to paying out-of-pocket for long term care services that are not covered by Medicare or insurance. One of the biggest fears many people have is spending all of their hard-earned assets to pay for care in their old age. Long term care insurance will help protect those assets by paying for long term care services that Medicare and health insurances don't cover. These services are considered "custodial" or "maintenance" rather than medical in nature. Ironically, these are the services that will keep mom or dad stable and, hopefully, in less need of "medical" services. Some of these services are companion care, personal care, assisted living facilities, and long term care facilities.

While long term care insurance may seem expensive at first, even if the yearly premium is $4000, remember that that amount (or a lot more) can be gobbled up in one month in a long term care facility.

Life Insurance

People usually buy life insurance to take care of burial expenses or to provide for a loved one when they are gone. However, don't discount this as a possible source of funds for care while your parent is living. Some policies have a cash surrender value that can be tapped into for care. As insurance commercials point out, life changes. Maybe that life insurance policy dad bought when he was worried about providing for his family if he died is needed now to pay for care. By the way, Medicaid usually considers life insurance with cash value as an asset.

WHO'S ON FIRST?

One last thing to consider when you are looking at these payment sources is the order in which these folks pay. Because all of these payment sources would really prefer that someone else foot the bill, when more than one payment source covers the same service a standard hierarchy falls into place. For the most part, your provider will take care of this, but it might help to understand what is going on behind the scenes. This is a diagram of the standard order:

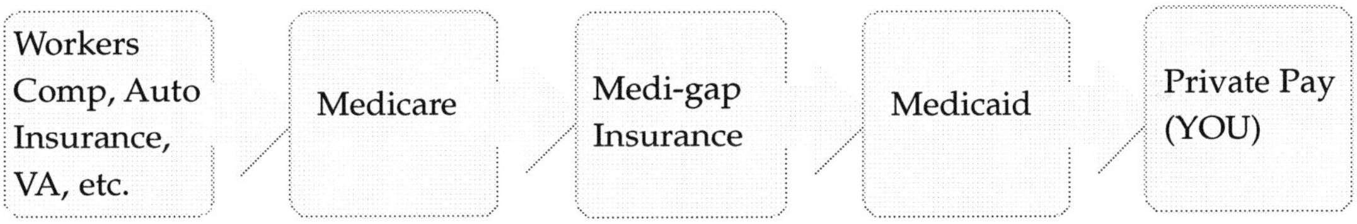
Workers Comp, Auto Insurance, VA, etc.
Medicare
Medi-gap Insurance
Medicaid
Private Pay (YOU)

The buck stops on private pay (which means you or your parents) but not before going through several other hoops. Each of these payment sources are going to produce paperwork showing what they have paid and what they will not cover. Keep all of this paperwork together in the files we talked about in Chapter Two. Since these folks all want to pay their piece in a specific order it often takes a long time for all of this to happen and the provider to get the total payment.

Here is an example of how the provider receives payment:

Your seventy-eight-year-old father suffers a broken right shoulder in a car accident. The medical portion of the car insurance should pay first for his right shoulder. However, he was on his way to physical therapy at an outpatient therapy clinic for the arthritis in his left knee. Medicare will continue to pay the therapist for the left knee while the car insurance pays for the right shoulder. However, Medicare only pays 80% of the therapy charges. Your father's Medi-gap insurance will pay the 20% less any deductible that the Medi-gap insurance requires. If your father is also eligible for Medicaid, in some states the Medicaid will cover the Medi-gap deductible. In addition, Medicaid will probably pay for his arthritis medication, except for the small co-pay that some states require on all prescriptions.

The outpatient physical therapy clinic will end up billing the following people:

1. The auto insurance for the right shoulder
2. Medicare for the left knee
3. Medi-gap insurance for the deductible and co-pay on the right knee
4. Medicaid for the Medi-gap deductible
5. Your father for the car insurance deductible (which might also be covered by Medicaid)

Now you know what all those folks in the billing office are doing: they are chasing down claims!

SIGNPOSTS IN THE MAZE

Now that you are seriously confused, it is time for a few words of encouragement. As patchwork as this system is, what you need to keep most in mind are those original three questions:

1. Is the person eligible for the payment source?
2. Is the service covered by the payment source?
3. Is the provider certified to accept the payment source?

Most of the other issues can and will be sorted out in the business office of your parent's provider. Despite the headlines about fraud, most providers are honestly trying to provide care within the framework of rules set down by the payment sources.

In the appendix you will find a list of websites and other contact information for payers and the folks who regulate them. These folks are there to answer your questions, so contact them. After all, in the final analysis your parents are the customers in this maze. While the customer might not always be right, the customer does have the right to an explanation.

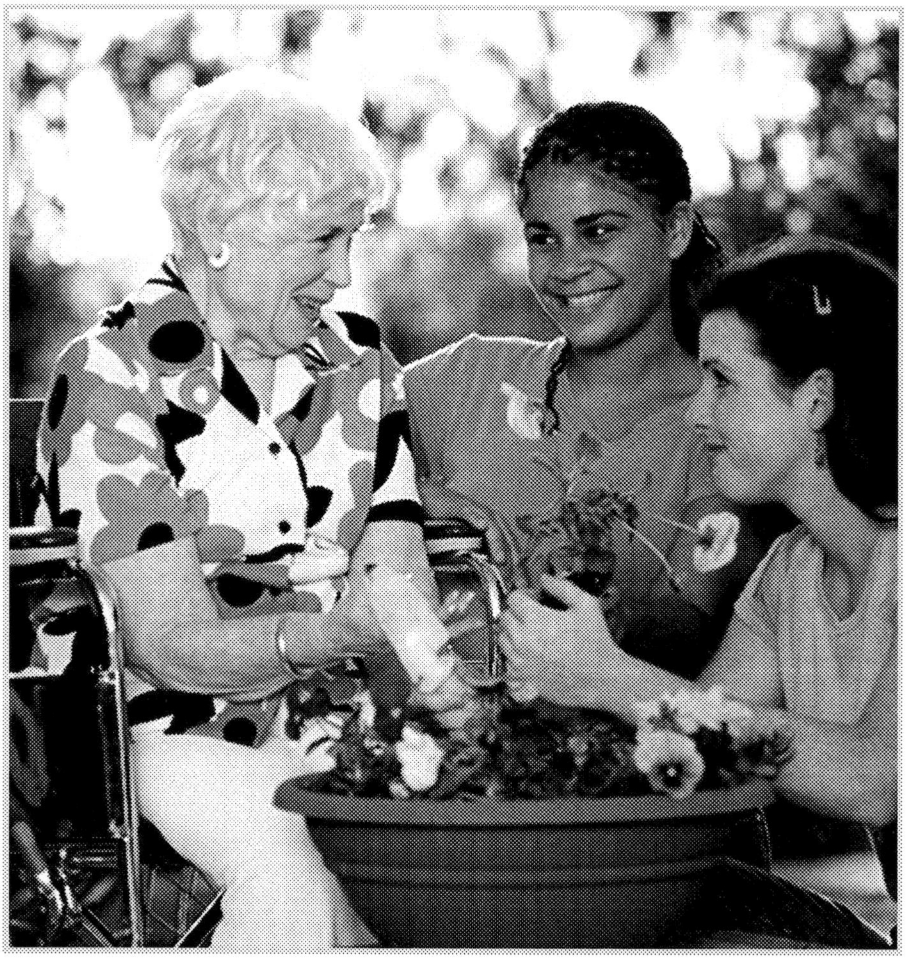

"...while juggling our own complex families and jobs, the idea of hiring people to help just makes sense..."

CHAPTER FIVE:

Helping Hands At Home

"Many hands make light work."
Anonymous

THE GOOD NEW DAYS

In 1980 I began my first job in elder care as a social worker at an eighty bed nursing facility. At that time, the county I lived in had seventy thousand people, one home health agency, two nursing facilities, and a small skilled unit at the county hospital. Each of the small towns in the county also had a senior citizens center offering congregate meals and social activities. At the nursing facility where I worked, we got our oxygen in big heavy tanks from a welding supply company and our medication from the local pharmacy. Wheelchairs and such were either ordered from a catalog or the local pharmacy. These services were typical of geriatric services across America.

Fast forward to 2004. Today this same county has one-hundred-twenty thousand people. It also has five home health agencies, five nursing facilities each with a skilled unit, five assisted living facilities, one retirement apartment complex, five companion care agencies, a rehab hospital, the county hospital, which is now the "regional medical center," and the senior citizens centers provide meals on wheels, congregate meals, and other activities. There are also six businesses selling oxygen and/or medical equipment in addition to the pharmacies. Senior services have grown exponentially as our population ages. If an area as isolated as San Juan County, New Mexico has all of these services, just think what might be in your neck of the woods.

One of the oldest myths about caregiving is that since mom took care of you, you are totally responsible for taking care of her. Think about this for a minute. As a child, did you go to school? Who was that person who stood in the front of the classroom and ruled most of your day for nine months per year? Unless you were home schooled, it was probably a professional teacher. What about Brownie leaders, Sunday school teachers, coaches, babysitters, and even your grandparents? If you are a mom yourself, you can probably add a few names to this list such as the Montessori director, the dance teacher, and your pediatrician. The concept that it takes a village to raise a child also holds true in senior care. The proliferation of services gives your folks a lot more options in where and how they wish to be cared for.

As an adult child, you may be the primary caregiver and doing just fine. Your caregiver role began gradually and became just one more facet of your life. You found yourself doing more of the driving for mom. Or, you got in the habit of cooking extra and taking meals over to your dad's house. For many families, this is just a normal part of family life. These families would be shocked if anyone even suggested they were doing anything special.

However, if you are moving past informal caregiving, these services may be just what you need to give your parents some support while maintaining your sanity.

THE HIRED GIRL

My mother was raised in a household that included her wheelchair-bound grandmother, who was paralyzed by a stroke. The family business was a cattle ranch, so in addition to a large extended family, there were always a few extra cowboys to feed. No wonder they hired a woman to help out in the house!

While my grandparents were not wealthy, the "hired girl" was a necessity of their life. Today, when we are faced with caring for our elderly parents while juggling our own complex families and jobs, the idea of hiring people to help just makes sense.

A lot has changed since my mother was a child in the 1930's. It was fairly simple for my grandparents to find a neighbor girl from a "good" family to come work for them. Wages were tight and there were very few jobs for women. Today, however, hiring someone to help with mom is a whole new world.

A CAST OF THOUSANDS

OK, maybe not quite thousands, but you will find that caring for mom and dad at home can require a lot of people. Even in this arena, providers have specialized. In fact, just arranging care can become so complicated that a new profession has emerged: the Geriatric Care Manager (GCM). The GCM is usually a social worker, counselor, or RN with specialized training in geriatrics. The GCM will assist you and your parents by assessing needs, developing a plan of care, and arranging services either in the home or in a facility. Especially if you live at a distance from mom or dad the GCM can help fill in the blank spaces in care as well as being your liaison to providers. The National Association of Professional Geriatric Care Managers is listed in the appendix.

Whether you are using a GCM or not, it is important to understand the differing roles of various caregivers. The first group listed below is of non-medical caregivers. This means that they cannot administer medications, change bandages, or provide other care that requires a licensed person. On the other hand, these are the folks who will take care of everything else—meals, companionship, housekeeping, laundry, errands, appointments, and on and on.

You will probably find that, even if your mom needs medical care, that there is still a place for the non-medical providers. One of the truths of senior care is that medical folks are so limited in time that they rely a great deal on non-medical folks to fill in the gaps. You may end up with more than one type of provider giving care to mom.

NON-MEDICAL CARE

THE FREEBIES (OR CLOSE TO IT)

In most communities, there are government and non-profit agencies to provide care for the elderly. AAA (Area Agency on Aging) operates many of these programs. Isn't it nice to know that some of your tax dollars are coming back home? Normally these agencies are free or low cost. Some examples of these are: the Senior Citizens Centers, RSVP, and Senior Companions. Usually these agencies are limited by their grants and funding sources to provide only specific duties for a set amount of time. For example, Senior Companions may send someone into the home for one to three hours per week. The companion can do light housework and companionship but not provide transportation or personal care.

Another service that falls in this area is Meals on Wheels. This program, usually available through your local Senior Citizen's Center, provides a hot meal to the home bound on a daily basis. Some programs provide meals seven days per week, while others only serve five days per week. Even if you use other services, Meals on Wheels is a good supplement.

PRO: Low cost, available in most areas

CON: Limited hours and duties

SUGGESTION: When looking for care, this is a good place to start. Just be sure you understand the scope of services provided by these programs, as they are often quite limited.

COMPANION CARE AGENCIES

A new growth field in our country is private agencies that provide "companion care" or "in-home non-medical care." While not yet available in all areas, the number of agencies is growing rapidly so there will probably be one in your neighborhood soon. Services provided include: meal preparation; housekeeping; laundry; some assistance with *ADLs*; transportation; and general companionship. The amount of time—from a few hours per week to live-in—depends only on your payment source. Payment is usually from long term care insurance or your own pocket.

Like all services, you need to check out the agency, using some of the questions below. One question that is particularly important to answer is whether the caregivers are employees of the agency or independent contractors. If the employee is an independent contractor, then you are actually making a contract with an individual not an agency. This can lead to all of the problems associated with private caregivers listed below.

PRO: more extensive hours available, staff is screened and supervised, and private agencies are normally the most flexible in terms of availability because they are not tied by grant money. The agency takes on all the employer responsibilities such as payroll, hiring/firing, taxes, insurances, worker's compensation, bonding, etc. They also take care of providing a substitute if the caregiver is absent. If you have ever had to cancel a business trip because the caregiver didn't show up, you will understand how important this is!

CON: More expensive than the government-sponsored programs.

SUGGESTIONS: Since this is still a new concept in many areas, check with your local Better Business Bureau or Chamber of Commerce for references.

MEDICAID PERSONAL CARE OPTION (PCO)

The name of this program may vary according to your state, so check with your state Medicaid program to see if this is available. The program is very similar to companion care agencies. In fact, some private companion care agencies also have a contract with the state Medicaid program for this option.

The big difference between this option and companion care agencies is that Medicaid pays for this program. This means two things for you:

1. Your parents must qualify for Medicaid
2. The program must comply with the Medicaid regulations regarding services, paperwork, and amount of time in the home

Under PCO programs, some states allow the client to hire their own caregivers with the Medicaid program picking up the tab. In these situations, you are responsible for hiring, firing, and finding your own replacements. Make sure you understand what is expected of you when you sign up.

PRO: Same as the companion care companies with the addition that Medicaid is paying for it.

CON: Hours and services are limited by the state Medicaid program. Under some client-directed programs, you can spend a great deal of time finding and supervising mom's caregivers.

QUESTIONS TO ASK

COMPANION CARE AGENCY/MEDICAID PCO

1. If your state requires licensure, is the agency licensed?
2. Do you have references from other clients?
3. Exactly what services will be you providing?
4. What training/experience do your caregivers have?
5. How do you supervise your caregivers?
6. Are your caregivers bonded?
7. What is the schedule?
8. How do I change the schedule?
9. What do I do if I have a problem with a caregiver?
10. Do you have an emergency phone number?
11. What are the financial arrangements?
12. Who owns your agency? Is it part of a larger organization?
13. Are your caregivers employees or independent contractors?
14. Do you carry Professional Liability Insurance?

PRIVATE CAREGIVERS

This is back to the old "hired girl" concept: find someone by running an ad or through a temp agency to take care of your parent. Many caregivers hired individually will live-in. Since the private caregiver is your employee, you have final say-so in their duties.

PRO: Within your budget, you have total flexibility. These folks are usually less expensive than using an agency.

CON: It is often difficult to find the right person. Since you are the employer, you are responsible for doing your own background checks, providing backup if the caregiver is absent, and paying the employer portion of taxes. Even more important, you are also taking on all of the liabilities of being an employer, including providing worker's compensation. If you chose not to provide state mandated worker's compensation, you are at great risk if your employee is injured. This is definitely a case of *caveat emptor.*

QUESTIONS TO ASK

PRIVATE CAREGIVERS

1. What references do you have from other clients?
2. What is your experience/background?
3. Do you have any certificates or training? If they have a CNA certificate, check with the registry at the state health department to see if it is still in effect.
4. Have you ever dealt with (Alzheimer's, cancer, etc.)?
5. What would you do if my mother had a medical emergency? Any other kind of emergency?
6. What notice would I have if you could not come in for the day? Can you arrange your own substitutes?
7. How do I contact you?
8. Are you bonded? Have you ever been convicted of a crime?
9. Do you have liability insurance and worker's compensation?
10. Exactly what services will you provide? Do you do personal care? Clean the house? Cook meals?
11. What are the financial arrangements? Remember that if you pay the caregiver over $600 per year, you must withhold taxes and you are responsible for the employer portion of the taxes.
12. Check also with your local adult protective services, Better Business Bureau, and any other references that you are given.

THE MEDICAL BAG

One of the big changes in medical care in the last twenty years has been that patients do not stay in the hospital for any length of time. For the elderly, with their slower recuperation times, this means that there is a need for more medical care at home. The good news is that a whole new world of post-acute care has sprung up like mushrooms after a rain. Even if you live in a remote area, you probably have a few medical options for taking care of mom at home.

All medical care must be ordered by the doctor and is for specific treatments or tasks. Medicare, health insurance, and Medicaid will usually pay for these specific treatments or tasks. This is great news, but the downside is that when these payment sources say that the treatment is not needed any longer, the agency must end their services.

One of the key factors in determining what is covered is the concept of medical necessity. In simple terms, medically necessary means that the attending physician has signed a statement that the particular treatment or service is needed because of the patient's diagnosis. If an item or treatment is considered to be for convenience only or the patient will not receive a medical benefit, then it is not medically necessary.

HOME HEALTH AGENCIES

A home health agency provides nurses, therapists, and home health aids to take care of your parent's medical needs such as monitoring medications, setting up IV's, and changing dressings on decubitus ulcers (bedsores). These agencies also provide physical, occupational, and speech therapies. A home health aid may be part of the team to assist with bathing and other "non-skilled" tasks.

The nurse in charge of your parent's care (often called the case manager) will organize this team. When the case manager, in consultation with your doctor, decides that the care is no longer medically necessary then home health will have to stop services. This can be especially frustrating in the area of therapies. Older people heal more slowly and have more problems with depression. This means that sometimes mom will just have a bad day and refuse to do her therapy. An occasional refusal will not end the therapy, but consistently refusing or not making any progress can cause therapy to be stopped.

By the way, the home health agencies understand this. They will usually try to continue services as long as possible. However, the reality is that continuing therapy or any other treatment paid for by Medicare when it is no longer deemed medically necessary is considered Medicare fraud. A reputable agency will not do it.

Home health agencies are licensed by the state and will usually be certified for Medicare and Medicaid as well as private insurance.

QUESTIONS TO ASK

HOME HEALTH CARE AGENCY

1. Is the agency licensed? Home Health Agencies are licensed by each state
2. May I see your last survey? Home Health Agencies are surveyed (inspected) by state health departments and/or JCAHO.
3. Exactly what services will you be providing?
4. Who will actually be caring for mom? Will she have the same nurse, therapist or home health aid each time?
5. When are visits scheduled? Will the visits be at the same time each week?
6. What do I do if I have a medical problem between visits?
7. What is your after-hours phone number if it differs from your daytime phone number?
8. What notification will I receive if services change?
9. When will services end?
10. What is your procedure if I have a complaint?
11. What are the financial arrangements?
12. Who owns your agency? Is it a part of a larger organization?

DURABLE MEDICAL EQUIPMENT PROVIDERS

When your parent needs equipment to make their life easier at home you will encounter the durable medical equipment (DME) folks. Often these folks also provide medical oxygen. If you need a hospital bed, wheelchair, or any other type of equipment your doctor will need to do certain paperwork so that the DME company can bill Medicare, Medicaid, or your insurance can pick up the tab.

Oxygen comes from a home respiratory business. Since this is considered a medicine, you must have a prescription for it just like an antibiotic. The prescription includes the rate of oxygen as liters per minute and the type of oxygen that the doctor prefers: concentrator, compressed gas, or liquid. While in years past, oxygen only came in big tanks so that folks were limited in their mobility, now oxygen is extremely portable.

While these companies will have a respiratory therapist on staff or as a consultant, most of the other folks working in these agencies are not medical people. This means the driver who delivers your oxygen can help you with information about the equipment, but that is all. Make sure that whoever sets up your equipment for the first time gives you a thorough explanation. Depending on the system, make sure you understand how to change tanks or refill the portable liquid oxygen systems. Also, make sure you understand what any alarms mean. Any questions about your actual treatment will need to be directed to the doctor.

HOSPICE

If your father's doctor states that he has less than six months to live, then he becomes eligible for hospice. Even if he lives longer, hospice will continue to provide care. Hospice provides nurses, social workers, counselors, and volunteers to help your father through the final months. Accepting hospice means that you have decided not to continue aggressive treatment, but still need supportive services such as pain management and physical care.

Medicare has developed a special Medicare Hospice benefit. When dad elects the Medicare Hospice benefit some of the rules regarding his Medicare change. The hospice organization becomes his case manager. If services not provided by the hospice agency are needed such as respite stays in the hospital or long term care facility, the hospice arranges and pays for these services. If he needs care for services because of a diagnosis that is not terminal, the payment reverts back to his original Medicare. For example, the hospice benefit pays for the pain medications for his cancer but if he breaks an arm, setting the arm will revert to original Medicare.

A good hospice agency can mean a better quality of life for your parent and the whole family through the final stages of life. However, there are a few things to make sure that you understand if you are considering hospice:

- Don't put off starting hospice until the last few days. Too often, people hesitate to call hospice until the last possible moment. The earlier you call, the more you and your dad will gain from hospice services.

- Hospice works with the family, it does not replace the family. Don't expect the hospice workers to totally take over your dad's care.
- As with all health-care workers, let the hospice agency know what you really need, especially if you are wearing out from the strain of daily care.

QUESTIONS TO ASK

HOSPICE

1. What special training does your staff have?
2. How often can I expect visits from the nurse, social worker, or other care providers?
3. Do you use volunteers? What do the volunteers do?
4. Who do I call in an emergency?
5. What happens if mom changes her mind about heroic measures?
6. I am finding this much more difficult than I thought it would be. How do you care for the family?
7. Is respite care available?
8. How do you coordinate with other services?

NOW I'VE GOT 'EM, WHAT DO I DO WITH 'EM?

Even with this cast of characters, it is important to understand that your parent (or you) is still in charge. Whether you are relying on outside folks to provide care or you are doing it all yourself, there are some basic issues that need to be addressed in any home. The next chapter will go into some details of daily care.

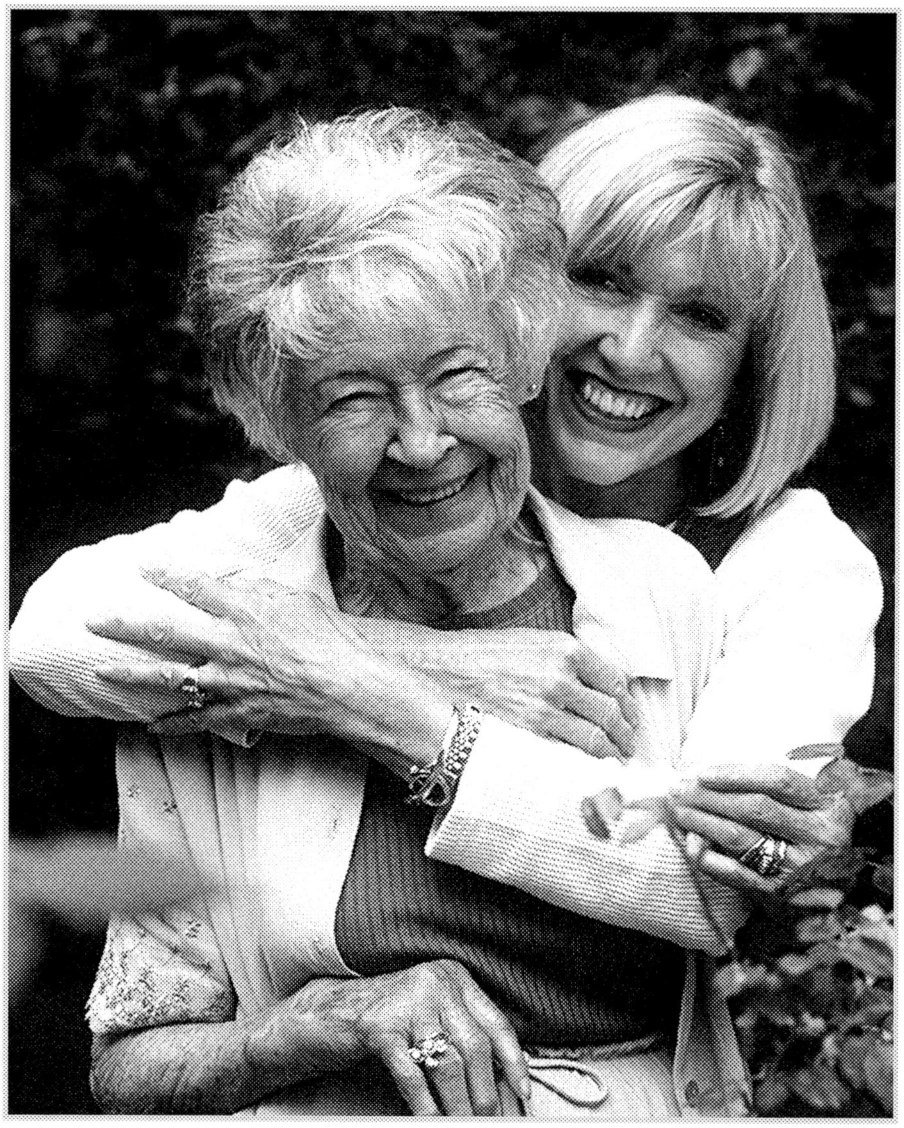

"...most people do not realize how very serious falls are for the elderly..."

CHAPTER SIX:

A Day in the Life of a Caregiver

"If I'd known I was going to live this long, I'd have taken better care of myself."

Eubie Blake

Every day you:

- Get out of bed
- Take a shower
- Get dressed
- Brush your teeth
- Style your hair
- Put on makeup (maybe not if you're a guy)
- Cook and eat a meal
- Wash the dishes
- Walk, stand, sit, kneel
- Hug your kids
- Hold hands with your spouse

and a dozen other things without ever thinking about the muscles that work to make this happen.

So what happens when one day you can't do these things? For many older folks and their families, this is where the real struggle lies. It isn't in the arena of big life and death medical decisions but in the day-to-day management of *Activities of Daily Living (ADL)*. Due to physical infirmity, an environment that doesn't fit present needs, or changes in mental status, the greatest challenge for the elderly is doing the basic things that most folks just take for granted. This chapter is all about the little (or not so little) things that we deal with everyday.

I'M FALLING FOR YOU

(From The Senior's Choice Fall Prevention Program)

When you were a child you probably fell a lot of times: off your bike, while playing sports, wrestling with your brother. Even as an adult, you may have tripped over the cat or slipped in the snow. Even though you may have been a little sore the next day, these falls were probably not a life changing experience. That is why most people do not realize how very serious falls are for the elderly. In fact, you might have become a caregiver because your parent had a serious fall.

The scope of this problem is so serious that Congress proposed the Elder Fall Prevention Act of 2002. The purpose of the act is to provide "A national approach to reducing elder falls which focuses on the daily life of senior citizens in residential, institutional, and community settings." Some of the statistics that were compiled in this act are frightening:

- Falls cause 70% of accidental deaths in people over seventy-five
- Falls cost $79 billion dollars in medical costs each year
- Falls cause 40% of all nursing home admissions
- One out of every three seniors living independently in their homes will experience a major fall each year
- 25% of seniors who suffer hip fractures die within one year

As the caregiver, what can you do to prevent falls and to make them less of a problem if they do occur?

The first thing you must do is to understand what causes falls and remove as many of these risks as possible. Some risk factors are not preventable: age; early onset menopause; and a family history of falls. Other risk factors are related to diagnosis: low blood pressure; Parkinson's disease; Alzheimer's; stroke; osteoarthritis; and vision deficits. Even with these factors in mind, there are many things you can do to prevent falls.

PREVENTING FALLS

One of the sad ironies of fall prevention is that the fear of falls is one of the factors that can cause them. When someone is weak, dizzy, or just can't see very well, they tend to remain seated the majority of the time. The problem with just sitting is that you become even weaker and so are more likely to fall. Therefore, the first thing to look at in fall prevention is maintaining the ability to walk and move independently. This means it is extremely important for the elderly to get a little exercise every day. Just a walk around the block or the mall will do wonders to prevent falls.

Making good use of the doctor's visit is also another good way to reduce the chance of falling. Make sure that your mom's doctor knows ALL of the medication she is taking, including those over the counter wonder drugs. Multiple medications can cause dizziness, drowsiness, and balance problems. Encourage dad to tell the doctor if he has had any weakness or other problems in his legs or feet.

While we are talking about doctors, it is a good idea for folks over sixty-five to have their hearing and vision checked annually. This will help prevent falls as well as flag any minor changes before they become big problems. By the way, if new glasses are prescribed allow a few days to adjust to the new prescription and keep those glasses clean.

Another overlooked cause of falls is as simple as how mom dresses. Does she wear loose, slick soled shoes or slippers? If she wears high heels, are they too high or are the heels worn around the edges? Worn shoes or slippers cause many falls, as do long nightgowns or robes with tie belts that drag the floor.

Falls also happen when folks don't think before reaching or bending. Like my mother's experience, standing on tables or chairs in order to reach overhead objects can cause a serious tumble. Likewise, reaching down to pick things up off the floor or from a low shelf can cause dad to become unbalanced. Try to have frequently used items in kitchens and bathrooms within easy reach.

Speaking of bathrooms, this is the number one room for falls. Consider adding grab bars to the walls near the toilet, shower, or bathtub. Other useful items are tub seats, hand-held showers, and non-skid tub mats.

The list of other adaptive devices includes walkers, canes, reachers (a tool for picking up items), elevated toilet seats, etc. If you see the need for these devices be sure to discuss it with your doctor. In some situations, Medicare will pay for adaptive devices if prescribed by the doctor.

HOME SAFE HOME

- Is lighting adequate? Poor vision is made worse by poor lighting. Consider nightlights for midnight trips to the bathroom or kitchen. Keep a flashlight by the bed for emergencies.
- Tack down or get rid of throw rugs. Look for tears in carpet or flooring.
- Stairs need sturdy handrails. Bright strips of tape can be added to the edge of each stair.
- Get rid of clutter in the walking path such as shoes, extension cords, and reading material. Keep pathways clear!
- Assess the furniture. Low or worn furniture can make it harder to stand up. Chairs with arms and back support are easier to get out of. A solid piece of furniture to hold onto while getting in and out of bed might be helpful.
- Pets are great companions. Just be aware that they can become mobile tripping hazards.

IF A FALL HAPPENS

Falls always seem to happen at the worst possible time, usually when someone is alone. So what should your mother do if she has a fall?

The first thing to do is to try to remain calm and not panic. The next step is to get help as quickly as possible. The length of time that a person is on the floor greatly influences their recovery from any injuries. Some folks get in the habit of carrying the telephone with them as they move around the house or yard.

Personal emergency response systems (PERS) are an excellent idea for anyone living alone or who has any risk factors for falls. These systems consist of a button that is worn on the wrist or neck and a telephone dialer that is attached to the house phone. When the button is pushed, the dialer calls a centralized phone center where an operator will notify a list of potential responders and/or call an ambulance. These systems are cheap insurance that mom won't lie on the ground waiting for help.

WHAT TO DO IF YOU FALL

If You Are Hurt--

- Don't try to get up since you could make it worse
- Move to a soft surface such as a carpet
- Keep warm using whatever is within reach to cover you
- If possible, move side to side to prevent pressure sores and/or hypothermia
- Move your arms and legs, if possible, to maintain body temperature

If You Are Not Hurt--

- As you fall, try to land on the padded areas of your side or buttocks
- Roll over on your stomach and attempt to get to hands and knees
- Crawl to a stable piece of furniture (bed, stool, chair without rollers or casters)
- Approach support from front and place both hands on the surface
- With both hands on support, place foot of stronger leg flat on the floor
- Lean forward as you begin to push yourself up with your hands while bringing your feet side-by-side
- Slowly turn and sit on the support
- Collect yourself before attempting to get up again

MOVE IT OR LOSE IT

Before we leave the subject of falls, I have just a few more comments about the whole arena of physical movement. One of the old myths about aging is that you need to slow down as you age. While nature might slow you down a little, too many folks take this natural slowing down to an unnatural extreme. For example, if dad was a runner all his life, he might find himself adding a few seconds to his best time. It does not mean he needs to give up running altogether, it just means that he needs to pace himself a little better. Retiring to the rocking chair will only allow those muscles he worked so hard to develop to atrophy until they will no longer do the job they were designed for. Therapists use the cliché "if you don't use it, you lose it" to describe this phenomena. No one ever slowed down the aging process by waiting it out in a rocking chair. In fact, studies repeatedly show that older folks who exercise regularly are healthier and happier. Arthritis and diabetes are just two conditions that tend to improve (or at least not worsen) when exercise is a part of daily life. So keep on moving!

IT'S SUPPERTIME!

In the play "You're a Good Man Charlie Brown" there is a truly wonderful moment where Snoopy sings the praises of the well-filled doggie dish at suppertime. With his increasingly frenzied singing and dancing, he extols the virtues of food. You know that Snoopy is going to relish every bite of that meal when it is put in front of him. But what happens when meals are no longer joyous events but, quite frankly, significant problems?

After falls, probably the issue that most often causes significant medical problems among the elderly is not eating. Most people know that proper nutrition is important at any age. There are countless books, magazines, websites, etc. devoted to different theories of exactly what constitutes good nutrition. But knowing that you need to eat right and doing it is not necessarily the same thing.

Eating problems in the elderly are usually in one or more of these areas:

- Getting food
- Eating food
- Specialized diets

If you are just becoming aware of issues with your parents, it might be difficult to realize that a major issue might be literally getting food on the table. In our society, getting food does not seem like it should be a problem. We live in the take-out nation. The grocery store is full of frozen dinners and other convenience foods so that getting a meal on the table can be as simple as heating something up in the microwave for a few minutes.

BUT, just because food is in the house does not mean it will be eaten. In doing home assessments, we always make a point of discussing food. Adult children often have great memories of mom's home cooking. When they are home for a visit, mom might make a special effort to cook old favorites or a visiting child might take mom out for a meal. If you happen to open the cabinets or the refrigerator it might seem full of food, just like you remember mom's kitchen.

Take a minute to look more closely at the contents of the cabinets and refrigerator. How current are the expiration dates? Are the frozen dinners iced over in the freezer? Are the little dabs of leftovers dried up in the margarine tubs? Just because food is in the house does not mean it is getting to the table.

This may be your first point of intervention. If you live nearby, dropping by at mealtimes to make sure that food is actually being consumed might be a start. Whether you use volunteer or paid companion care, schedule your caregivers to be in the house during mealtime.

Use your medical resources to make sure there is not a physical reason why mom never seems hungry. Is she on a medication that is suppressing her appetite? Does she have dental problems such as loose dentures or sores in her mouth?

Of course, there are also social reasons why older people stop eating. Too often you hear, "it's too much work to cook for one," "nothing tastes good," or "I'm not really hungry."

"It's too much work to cook for one" syndrome can sometimes be addressed by using those community resources of Senior Citizen Centers. The advantage of going to the Senior Center for meals is that it also takes care of the message, "I don't like eating alone." Most centers encourage a convivial atmosphere where friendships are formed over chicken noodle casserole. If you live in the same community, getting together with your parents for a regular weekly meal can serve the same purpose. And sending home the leftovers with mom or dad can take care of the next meal, too.

The problem with any take-out food, whether it comes from your kitchen, Meals on Wheels, or the grocery store deli, is that it loses some of the taste on the way to your dad's house. One of the best things you can do to make these meals more appetizing is to put them on your own china and give them a few seconds in the microwave.

"Nothing tastes good" has to do with the fact that our taste buds change as we age. Like the other senses, the sense of taste tends to diminish with age. Add to that the odd metallic taste that certain medicines have, it's no wonder that nothing tastes like mom remembers. This also explains why you will see folks salting their food until it glistens or adding a couple extra packets of sugar to their coffee or tea. Making foods flavorful by using marinades, herbs, or sauces might help this.

Also, make sure that dad goes to the dentist regularly for checkups. If he wears dentures, notice if they are loose or ask if he has rubbed sores. Poor teeth, sore gums, or loose dentures can all cause dad to not want to bother with food.

THE SAUERKRAUT QUESTION

I worked for a few years in a facility in Nebraska. For our residents with German and Slavic roots, sauerkraut was a staple. However, the daughter of a resident in New Mexico was very angry when sauerkraut appeared on the facility menu.

"Don't you know old people can't eat gassy things like sauerkraut!" she demanded.

A few days later at a family meeting in the same facility, one of the primary concerns was the fact that the facility needed to serve Mexican food more often. In fact, several families regularly brought in their own homemade chili for their loved ones because ours was not hot enough!

The area where I now work borders the Navajo reservation. Blue corn meal mush and mutton stew are on the menu of all the facilities in the area. These are not my personal favorites (though I love Navajo tacos). I have learned, however, that blue corn meal mush can work miracles if a frail elderly Navajo man or woman refuses to eat.

All of us have "comfort foods" that make us feel better. Remember the foods on your mother's table when you were a child? Even if they are no longer your favorites, they might just be the key to get dad eating again.

SPECIALIZED DIETS

The doctor may suggest that your father follow a specific diet, especially if he has a diagnosis such as diabetes, high blood pressure, or end stage renal disease. The good news is that in the last few years, many of these diets have become much less restrictive. The bad news is that many people still balk at the idea of ANYONE restricting their diet. Many organizations that focus on diseases have extensive advice on managing these diets. Some of their websites are listed in the resource listing in the appendix.

OTHER FOOD ISSUES

The daughter in the above story did have a point: sometimes the issues are of the heartburn, bloating variety. If they are, then avoid the foods that cause this. Try numerous small meals throughout the day, and stick to bland low fat foods.

Another major concern is the constipation/diarrhea syndrome. If your parent is having problems in this area first talk to the doctor. Be sure to tell the doctor about any over the counter laxatives or antidiarrhetics your parent is taking. Sometimes bowel problems are caused by medication or people get in the habit of using a lot of over the counter laxatives to get relief. Then they start taking something else to counter the laxatives. Before you know it, what was a simple problem has become very complex. Also, look at natural ways to deal with these issues. Everyone is more regular if they eat high-fiber foods, drink LOTS of liquids, and exercise daily.

THE BEAUTY QUEEN

Like the list at the beginning of this chapter suggests, every day you do a lot of routine activities in the area of general hygiene. We go through these daily chores because most of us feel better if we are clean. However, remember last winter when you had the flu? Remember how the very thought of a shower just seemed to take too much energy? Sometimes that's the way it feels for the elderly. Combine this with the very real fear of a fall in the bathroom and it is easy to see why personal hygiene can begin to suffer.

It is very hard to admit that mom isn't bathing as often as needed. But, like most problems in life the first step is to admit there is a problem. Is mom not bathing because she is afraid of slipping in the shower? Go back to the section on falls. Make sure the bathroom is equipped with all of the safety equipment such as grab bars and shower bench. Even if she is still independent, it might also be a good idea to offer for someone to be in the house while she showers, just in case she needs to call for help.

Set up a regular beauty shop appointment where mom can have her hair and nails done. Not only will this take care of the hygiene issue, it will also give her a chance to catch up on the gossip at the local beauty shop. Beauty shop therapy is good for the spirit as well as the hair!

THE SKIN GAME

Older skin tends to be dryer than younger skin. This is why it is often a good idea not to shower daily. A hot daily shower will dry out the skin and leave it rough and reddened. Use a moisturizing soap or body wash and plenty of lotion after the shower. Dry skin is another reason why older people need to be encouraged to drink lots of fluids.

One of the biggest threats to an older person with poor circulation is the possibility of skin breakdown that can progress to decubitus ulcers, otherwise known as bedsores. These are usually caused by a bony area (heels, hip bones, tailbone, etc.) pressing down on a small area of the skin, which prevents blood circulation in the area, causing the skin to die. Like falls, the true risk of decubitus ulcers is usually underestimated. These sores can be very difficult to heal and can be life-threatening. The best way to deal with skin breakdown is to try to prevent it from happening in the first place.

- Keep the skin clean and dry, especially in skin folds.
- Make sure the bed linens are clean, dry, and wrinkle free.
- Move around so that blood circulation is maintained. This means that the older person should change positions at least every two hours, even while in bed.
- Massage moisturizing lotion into reddened areas. Massaging will encourage the blood to circulate and the lotion will help keep the skin supple.
- Don't sit or lay on hard surfaces. There is a huge variety of pressure reducing pads and cushions on the market but all of them work by conforming to the body and spreading out the pressure area.
- Make sure that circulation is not cut off by tight clothing or shoes. Especially watch for tight elastic in socks or stockings.

THOSE WONDERFUL SENSES

If you wear glasses, have you ever had to go a day without them? Do you find yourself not having arms quite long enough to get the newspaper to the point you can read it? Have you ever struggled to hear someone who insisted on using a speaker phone from across the room? Do you remember that awful head cold when your head seemed stuffed with cotton and nothing tasted or smelled right? Then you might have experienced just a little of what happens to your senses as you age. All of the senses that keep you in touch with the world are affected by aging. This is why it is so extremely important to make sure that your parents have their vision and hearing checked at least once a year.

Hearing loss is often very gradual and may be disguised by other problems. If dad doesn't hear well, he may just turn up the volume on the TV or withdraw from conversation. He may seem depressed or frustrated. Sometimes caregivers start suspecting dementia when the real problem is that dad cannot hear well enough to follow the conversation so he interrupts with comments that don't appear relevant.

The good news about hearing and vision loss is that there have been many medical advances in treating these common problems. Hearing aids are less obtrusive and produce clearer sound than a generation ago. Cataract surgery is now a simple outpatient procedure. Even bifocals are now disguised so that no one else has to know you are wearing them.

Keeping those senses as sharp as possible will keep dad in the game a lot longer.

THE MOST IMPORTANT SENSE OF ALL

When you hold a baby, you may have an overwhelming urge to cuddle and caress that incredible smooth soft skin. Parents nuzzle, stroke, and kiss little toes and tummies. It is almost as if we are programmed to want to touch babies. That's a good thing, because even scientists agree that babies need a certain amount of touch to survive.

So what happens to old people? Do they lose the need to touch just as their skin loses the moisture and elasticity of youth? Of course not. Everyone needs to be touched, but not everyone gets touched. Just as there is something that draws us to touching babies, there seems to be something that makes people tend to shy away from touching old folks.

From holding hands and rubbing shoulders, to hugging and kissing, every person needs touch, no matter their age. Touch is one of the last senses we lose. So keep touching, keep holding hands, and keep on hugging. Your touch may be the most important experience of your mom's day.

LAST THOUGHTS

This chapter is just a brief glimpse of the daily issues of caring for your parent with declining physical abilities. Many of these same issues affect folks when the decline is mental. However, there are often different and very difficult challenges when the changes are mental. Therefore,

Chapter Seven will focus on what to do when the person you knew becomes another person entirely.

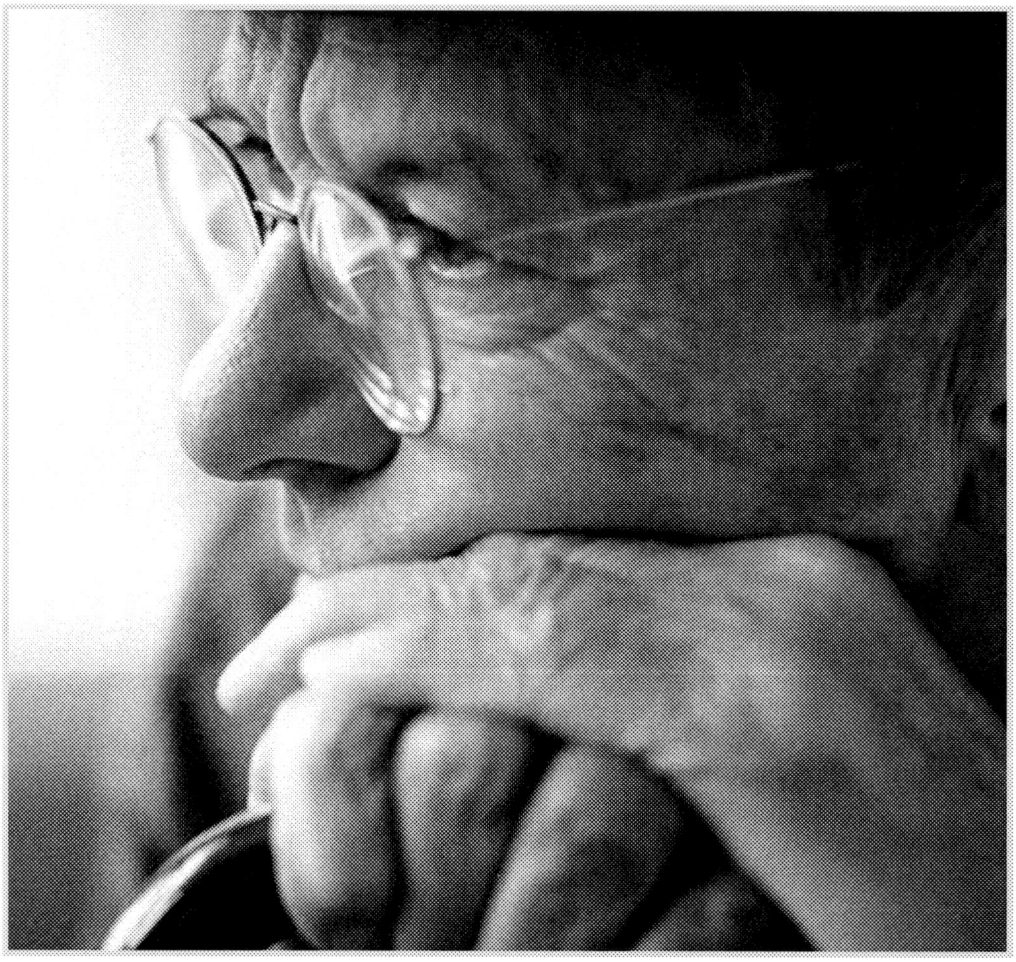

"...the issue of safety. With the loss of judgment that occurs with dementia comes a loss of safety awareness..."

CHAPTER SEVEN:

An Altered State of Reality

> *"How old would you be if you didn't know when you were born?"*
>
> *Anonymous*

Meet my friend, Pearl. Years ago Pearl was a high school math teacher. She was the kind of teacher that could make even algebra accessible. Pearl and her husband, Homer, raised two daughters and a son. All three children went to college and entered careers of their own. When Pearl and Homer retired, they bought an RV. The next few years of their lives they gleefully filled in a sticker map of the country as they traveled to most of the western states. However, the last few years the RV hasn't moved much. Pearl can't seem to get her act together to pack it.

Homer doesn't want to worry the kids, but he is starting to wonder who is losing their mind: Pearl or himself. The other night, he woke up and Pearl wasn't in the house. He finally found her outside knocking on the door of the RV. She was standing in a snowdrift in her nightgown and slippers; her thin legs were blue from the cold. When he tried to take her back inside, she didn't seem to know him at first. Then Pearl accused Homer of having an affair with "the woman" living in the RV.

WHAT IS DEMENTIA?

According to the Alzheimer's Association:

"Dementia is a loss of mental function in two or more areas such as language, memory, visual and spatial abilities, or judgment severe enough to interfere with daily life. Dementia itself is not a disease but a broader set of symptoms that accompanies certain diseases or physical conditions." *Alzheimer's Disease and Related Dementias Fact Sheet*

In other words, dementia is the result of a disease process, not the cause. What does that mean if you are the person dealing with a family member who is suddenly exhibiting some rather bizarre behavior? It means that you should be taking your mom, dad, husband, or wife to the doctor for a complete physical as soon as possible.

Many folks hold the mistaken belief that these behaviors prove that mom is "going crazy" or dad is just "getting senile" like all old folks do. It is embarrassing to admit that your husband needs you to lead him to the bathroom. Or, maybe your wife is fine, but you are the one getting forgetful. And the doctor can't do anything about a little forgetfulness anyway.

WRONG! Some of the causes of dementia are reversible with treatment. These include depression, acute illness, metabolic changes, and certain medications. Other dementias are part of a chronic disease process, but some of the progression of the disease can be reduced with treatment. For example, multi-infarct or vascular dementia is caused by multiple small strokes. Treating the high blood pressure or vascular risks that causes the strokes can prevent further mental as well as physical deterioration. Other diseases that can produce dementia symptoms are Parkinson's disease, Huntington's disease, Creutzfeldt-Jakob disease, Pick's disease, and Lewy body dementia.

WHAT ABOUT ALZHEIMER'S?

The number one cause of dementia symptoms is Alzheimer's disease. Alzheimer's disease affects 4 million Americans, including Pearl. Alzheimer's is a progressive disease. That means Pearl didn't just wake up one morning with it. There are recognizable stages of the disease process that usually begin quite subtly. By the time others notice the changes in behavior, the disease may have been progressing for a long time. Over months and years, the Alzheimer's patient will gradually lose the ability to remember, think, and reason. In the final stages of the disease Pearl will not only lose her mental abilities but her physical ones also. It is almost as if the brain is working in reverse losing higher functions first and then working it's way backwards to those first motor skills we learn as babies.

New medications focus on slowing the disease progression while research continues for vaccinations or other methods to prevent the disease. Since there is no cure at this time, other medical interventions focus on treating symptoms like anxiety, depression, and sleeplessness. Pearl will probably also be more susceptible to other problems such as urinary tract infections and falls. Homer and the family will need to watch for physical changes, because Pearl will not always be able to say where it hurts. A routine visit to the doctor will be extremely important to keep Pearl as healthy as possible.

LIVING WITH DEMENTIA

One way that caring for a loved one with dementia differs from caring for a loved one with a physical condition, such as a broken leg, is the emotional toll it takes on the caregiver. Especially in the early stages, the person with dementia often appears to be totally lucid and in control. Therefore, when there is a lapse in judgment or a slightly unusual reaction to a situation, the caregiver will question his or her own judgment or behavior. The caregiver will think, "My wife isn't crazy, maybe I am!" or "Maybe he didn't leave his wallet in the freezer, I did."

Other folks may also perceive the caregiver as creating a problem where none exists. I remember a daughter telling me about calls from her mother's friends accusing her of trying to "put your mother away." What the friends had not seen, because the mother was still socially appropriate at times, was the dangerous behaviors such as leaving the stove on and wandering. The mother was also calling the daughter ten to twenty times per day often in tears.

Since dementia does not cause physical changes, (at least until the very late stages) it is hard for folks to understand what the caregiver is really dealing with. It is easy for outsiders to miss the real problems.

The next most important step is to arm yourself with information and resources to help guide you through the stages to come. The best resource that I have found is the Alzheimer's Association. These folks have an incredible amount of information about how the disease progresses and suggestions for dealing with each step. Equally important, most local chapters also sponsor support groups for the family. If you do nothing else for yourself, go to one of these support groups.

KEEPING IT SAFE

Many of the issues discussed in the last chapter will also apply if dad has dementia. For example, he may be at a higher risk for falls because he is less aware of risky behavior and has reduced motor skills. He may also forget to eat or bathe while insisting that he just ate a big breakfast and had a shower first thing in the morning.

In addition to the issues mentioned before, though, are some specific issues that are likely to become problems. The most important of these is the issue of safety. With the loss of judgment that occurs with dementia comes a loss of safety awareness.

Take a quick tour of dad's living environment for unsafe items, such as unlocked cleaning fluids, sharp knives left in drawers, or guns. It is truly amazing how clever someone with dementia can be about finding the one thing in the house that you would not want him to handle. While you're touring, check for tripping hazards.

One of the first safety issues that you may confront is the issue of driving. Let your doctor be your guide on this issue. Many families assume that since dad still knows the way to the grocery store and the barbershop it is all right for him to drive. But what happens if something unexpected happens on the route such as road construction or a child running into the street? Would dad have the ability to cope with these abrupt changes? Discuss this issue frankly with the doctor. If the doctor says it is time to stop driving, then let him be the one to tell dad. Sometimes hearing this news from a professional is easier to take than from the kid you taught to drive.

Another safety issue is the wandering behavior that is typical of dementia. Many folks will start pacing or wandering around the house and outside. Wandering sometimes gets worse when there is pain or discomfort from a physical condition such as a urinary tract infection or just needing to go to the bathroom, but for many dementia patients it is just a part of the condition.

The real danger with wandering is an unsafe environment or the fear that mom may get lost. This is the time to install hooks high up on doors that open onto busy streets or down basement stairs. Make sure that mom wears an ID bracelet. The Alzheimer's Association also has a program called *SafeReturn* that may be of assistance.

I'M TALKING BUT YOU'RE NOT HEARING

Communicating with mom also becomes a problem as the condition progresses. For folks with dementia one of the key problems is too much information coming in too quickly to process. Therefore, the key is to reduce the amount of information by speaking slower, in shorter sentences, and not introducing too many concepts at once. Also, look at background distractions, like the TV that is always turned on to CNN or the stereo in the background.

If mom insists that she has already had breakfast, don't argue. I have never known anyone to win an argument with a dementia patient. Either change the subject or try to listen between the lines. If someone is asking when the next meal is, maybe they are just hungry.

Over time, as the dementia progresses, mom may lose her ability to speak. It is important to still talk to mom, whether she responds or not. Just the sound of your voice and the touch of your hand will remind her that someone cares about her. That is really the most important thing to communicate.

WHEN THE TIME COMES

Since dementia is progressive, one of the real issues many families face is when home is no longer safe. Refer to the questions in Chapter Two again if you are struggling with this issue. If living alone is no longer an acceptable risk, this may be the time to explore adult daycare, move dad into your home, or consider a congregate setting such as an assisted living facility or nursing home. The next bend in the zone is homes away from home.

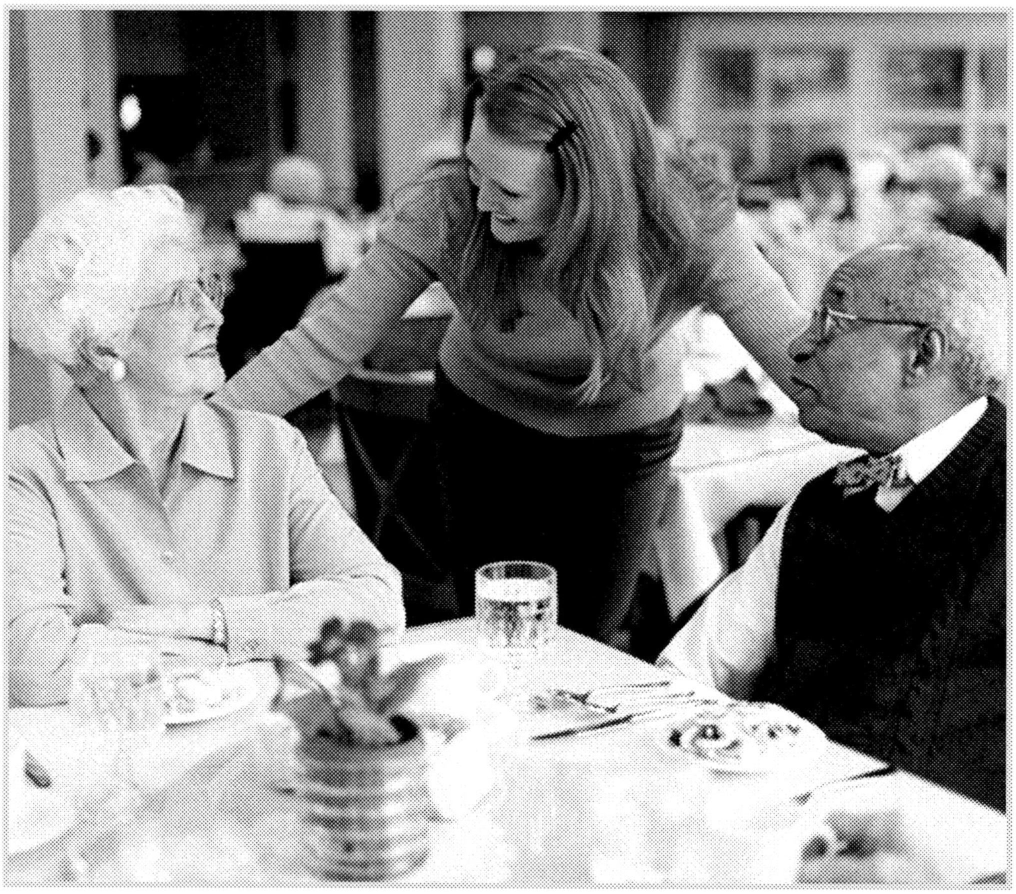

"...assisted living facilities usually include meals, assistance with personal care, some social activities, and staff available to supervise and help mom around the clock..."

CHAPTER EIGHT:

Homes Away from Homes

"Home is where the heart is and hence a moveable feast."

Angela Carter

WHEN HOME IS NO LONGER THE ANSWER

No one goes through life saying, "I can't wait to go to a nursing home," but then again I don't know very many people who really want to do surgery on the kitchen table. That is why we go to hospitals for surgery. For some of the same reasons, mom or dad's failing physical or mental health may make a move outside the home a necessity.

If you have picked up a senior newspaper or magazine recently, you have probably seen ads for the various homes away from home. The ads look more like they are advertising a country club than care for your mom. Many of the ads show a smiling white haired person and talk about quality care. The lady in the ad probably looks better than your mother, who may be lying in a hospital bed down the hall. Don't let these ads confuse you. Like all advertising, these ads are intended to sell the sizzle. This chapter is about the steak behind the sizzle.

When trying to find the right place for mom, consider first how much help she needs as well as what kind of help. Is she in the middle stages of dementia, is she recuperating from an injury so that rehab is the primary goal, or is she looking for a lifestyle change with lots of opportunities for socialization? Then look at which facilities offer the level of care that will best meet her needs. We are going to do a quick tour of several levels of care to give you a snapshot of what is available in practical terms.

SUN CITY OR BUST!

For many folks, the first move away from home is into a retirement community. So, what exactly is a retirement community?

Some retirement communities are like the pictures you see in the ads—the condo on the edge of the golf course with white haired folks riding to the grocery store in their golf carts. At the other end of the spectrum are efficiency-sized apartments with supportive services. In general, retirement communities provide congregate housing for folks over a certain age (fifty-five to sixty-five is the low range) that is structurally designed to accommodate older people.

Many retirement communities are on the same campus (or "village") as a skilled nursing facility or assisted living facility. Bringing together a variety of living arrangements and services together in one location keeps mom within an organization's system. This can be extremely helpful to mom or dad as they don't have to go far when their needs change due to illness, aging in place, or recovery.

The services provided in the independent living apartments or condos usually focus on the building: maintenance and yard work. Other services are more social: congregate dining (often in a restaurant type atmosphere) and activities such as exercise programs, a golf course, swimming pool, or club house. This can be a great environment for someone needing companionship and someone else to mow the grass.

If dad becomes sick or just needs more help, these communities can usually arrange a home health agency to come into their apartment or condo. However, if dad continues to need more help, the retirement community may suggest that it is time to consider moving into an assisted living facility or nursing home within the village.

The Price Tag

Your mom or dad normally pays the charges for independent living communities privately. HUD-sponsored senior housing projects are an exception to this rule. These projects can actually be on the same campus as private pay independent living, assisted living, and/or a nursing home, but the rules are very different.

HUD projects are aimed at low income tenants. While there are a lot of ins and outs to qualifying for these apartments, the bottom line is that your mom's income must be below a certain level. HUD senior apartments are usually small with a few amenities such as laundry room, meeting room, and a manager on site.

On the other end of the economic scale are the plush senior condos you see in the glossy ads. Payment for these retirement communities generally fall into two areas:

- Buy-in
- Pay as you go

In a buy-in situation mom buys her condo or apartment in the retirement community, usually for a significant amount of money. Once she has bought her condo or apartment, the organization will charge a monthly service fee for items such as utilities, maintenance, meals in the dining room, clubhouse activities, and an emergency call system. When mom moves out, her condo or apartment will be re-sold to another person by the sponsoring organization. This means that she should receive some of her money back, though the sum is usually pro-rated by the amount of time she lived in the apartment.

Since the buy-in is specific to the unit, it does not usually include assisted living or skilled nursing facilities even if these facilities are available on the same campus. Occasionally, as a marketing incentive, the organization will throw in a set number of nights per year in these other levels of care.

Continuing care retirement communities (CCRC) are similar to buy-ins. The difference is that you buy into a community that includes several levels of care. The idea is that mom will be taken care of for the rest of her life for a hefty upfront fee and monthly payments. Since these are such all inclusive arrangements, make sure that you fully understand all contracts and extra charges.

Pay as you go means that there is only a nominal up front move-in fee, like first and last month's rent, and you pay a monthly rental for the apartment or condo and associated services. These work much like any other lease.

QUESTIONS TO ASK

RETIREMENT COMMUNITIES/INDEPENDENT LIVING

1. What amenities are included in the regular charges?
   a. Housekeeping/laundry
   b. Yard maintenance
   c. Congregate meals
   d. Emergency call
2. What amenities are not included?
3. Is there on-site management?
4. What do you do in an emergency?
5. If my dad started needing more assistance, must he move or could arrangements be made for this assistance in his apartment?
6. Is there another level of care on site, such as a skilled facility or assisted living facility? What is your relationship?
7. What are the financial arrangements? How does the contract work?
8. Who owns the retirement community?
9. Can I visit with some of the folks who live here? Do they like it here?

ASSISTED WHAT?

One of the newer concepts in the long term care industry is the assisted living facility. Many folks who would not even consider admission to a nursing home are attracted to this new idea. Some of those glossy ads showing happy people are for assisted living facilities.

Assisted-living facilities (ALFs) fall in the gray area between independent living and the nursing home. Some assisted-living facilities look and feel much like retirement communities with a few added services while others tend toward being "nursing home junior." This is because there are no national regulations for this level of care. Instead, each state has decided what assisted living means under their jurisdiction. This has created a hodgepodge of differing communities defining themselves as assisted living facilities. Even the name for the facility can change: assisted living facility, board and care home, adult residential care facility.

In general, an assisted-living facility provides supportive services to seniors or the disabled in a residential setting. Some senior professionals refer to this as the "social model" of care. This is to differentiate it from skilled nursing facilities (SNFs), which are considered to be a "medical model." Services at assisted living facilities usually include meals, assistance with personal care, some social activities, and staff available to supervise and help mom around the clock.

In the medical care arena, most state regulations require that there is a nurse on staff or as a consultant. Usually only large facilities actually have a nurse on staff. Most of the smaller facilities arrange for a nurse to visit weekly or monthly. The staff responsible for day-to-day care is comprised of "resident assistants" workers who have had some training in personal care, safety, CPR, and related issues. The resident assistants may assist mom with medications, but not administer them. If your mother needs therapy or more intensive nursing care, most assisted living facilities will help you arrange a home health agency to provide these services, just like they would in your mother's home.

Since assisted-living facilities are on the social model, they work best for mom if she just needs help with meals, personal care, and someone generally around for visiting and supervision. However, if mom has extensive medical needs the assisted-living facility might not be able to provide the level of care that she requires. Some assisted-living facilities have developed special programs for folks with Alzheimer's or other special needs. The information listed under "Questions to Ask, Alzheimer's/Dementia Care" is appropriate for assisted-living facilities as well as skilled nursing facilities.

The Price Tag

The lack of cohesive regulations has also made paying for an assisted living more confusing. Medicare does not pay for assisted living facilities at all. In some states, Medicaid will pay for assisted living facilities. If mom is eligible for Medicaid, ask your Medicaid caseworker if this is a covered service in your state. Also, ask which assisted living facilities in your area accept

Medicaid. Many assisted living facilities have chosen not to participate in the Medicaid program because reimbursement rates are often quite low.

QUESTIONS TO ASK

ASSISTED LIVING FACILITIES

1. Is the facility licensed?
2. May I see the last state survey?
3. What is your ratio of resident assistants to residents during the day? At night?
4. How are your resident assistants trained and supervised?
5. Do you have a nurse on staff or on call? How many hours per day or week is the nurse on-site?
6. What are your emergency procedures?
7. Are special diets (such as diabetic or low sodium) available? Try to eat a meal in the dining room and ask your tablemates what they think of the food.
8. What recreational activities are provided? Are these at the facility or do you take residents to community activities?
9. Do you provide transportation to medical appointments? Some states only require that access to transportation be provided which could consist of a list of taxi phone numbers.
10. Do you have a beauty/barber shop? What is available if the facility does not have one?
11. How does mom get mail, phone calls, etc.?
12. What are your limitations on care? If mom needs assistance transferring to a wheelchair or starts wandering will she need to leave? What if she needs insulin injections? Wound care? Pain management? Feeding tube?

13. Who owns the facility?
14. Are there other levels of care available on the same campus?
15. What happens if mom is gone for a few days such as vacation, hospitalization, etc.? Is her room held at a lower rate?
16. Do you provide the furniture or does mom bring in her own furniture from home? Do you have any limitations?
17. What are the financial arrangements? Are there extra charges for more assistance? Do you accept long term care insurance?

THE NEW NURSING HOME

Back in the dark ages of 1980, when I began my career in long term care, some of my friends and family thought I was crazy to even consider working in a nursing home. After all, nursing homes are dark dreary places where old people are sent to die.

To the surprise of the naysayers, the first facility I worked in was only a few years old at the time, was bright and sunny, and I met some truly wonderful people there. Many of the residents were folks who just could not make it at home any more but they were still part of a community: planning an annual bazaar, winning ribbons at the county fair, and voicing their opinion about the food. In fact, in many ways this facility had more in common with today's assisted living facility than with the new skilled nursing facility.

Long term care facilities have changed a lot since 1980. In the late 1980's OBRA '87 and it's companion, OBRA '89, set off an atomic bomb in the nursing home industry creating new requirements for staffing, training, services, assessment and other issues. While this was the first major change, many others followed, including changes in how Medicare pays for skilled nursing care. If you have not visited a nursing home since 1987 or your only image is from TV and movies, you will probably be surprised. In fact, one of the issues in the industry is that professionals no longer call these facilities nursing homes. The correct term now is skilled nursing facilities (SNF).

When Long Term Care Is Short Term

One of the significant changes that came about since 1987 is the expansion of short term/long term care. As hospital stays decreased in length, the need for more intensive post-acute care increased. For example, twenty years ago if your mom had broken her hip, she may have stayed in the hospital for a month or more to recuperate. Now, however, Medicare will only pay for a limited hospital stay: just long enough to have surgery, stabilize, and begin therapy. Within a few days mom will be discharged. One of her options will be the skilled nursing facility.

At the skilled facility, mom will receive physical therapy as her hip heals. Occupational and speech therapy will also be available. A nurse will be responsible for her care, including administering all medications, monitoring her healing incision, and providing any other medical needs. All of this will be according to orders from her doctor. Certified nursing assistants (CNAs) will be responsible for helping her dress and undress, take a shower, and any other assistance she needs with activities of daily living.

If there aren't many complications, mom will probably be in the skilled nursing facility for one to two months. Then it will be time for her to go home. Her doctor may order home health to continue some of the therapy at home.

The Price Tag

Medicare usually pays for this kind of short term placement. Medicare has some basic guidelines for when they pay for skilled care:

- Mom must have been in the hospital for at least three days before being admitted to the SNF (if mom goes home from the hospital first, she has a window of thirty days to be admitted to the SNF)
- Mom must need a daily skilled service such as therapy or skilled nursing care such as sterile dressing changes, IVs, stabilizing medication regimes, etc.

Medicare will pay 100% of the charges for the first twenty days. After that, there will be a co-pay, which mom's Medi-gap policy or Medicaid will usually cover. This co-pay is currently over $100 per day and increases every year. Medicare totally stops paying after 100 days or whenever mom no longer needs daily skilled services.

The facility will keep track of mom's need for skilled services and the number of days. It is a good idea to ask periodically what skilled services mom is receiving and how soon they will end. Don't ever assume that she will stay the full 100 days.

Longer Long Term Care

What happens, though, if dad has a chronic condition necessitating long term twenty-four hour medical care? For example, what if he has a serious stroke that leaves him unable to function enough to go home even after extensive therapy? Or he has a combination of diagnosis such as Parkinson's, COPD, and diabetes?

That is what the rest of the skilled nursing facility is all about: taking care of folks with chronic long term conditions that require around the clock care. Since OBRA '87, skilled nursing facilities are required to have nurses on duty twenty-four hours per day to provide medical care and supervision. As above, CNAs will help dad with grooming, dressing, and other activities of daily living. If the doctor orders therapies, special diets, or other treatments such as wound care or oxygen therapy, these will also be provided by the facility. Skilled nursing facilities also go beyond medical care with activities, social services, and amenities such as beauty/barber shops.

During dad's long term stay, Medicare will pay for specific items such as therapies that are considered medically necessary, certain supplies, and very little else. Daily charges for dad's care will be paid by Medicaid, long term care insurance, or you.

What's So Special About Special Care?

Specialty units are one of the new and improved areas of skilled nursing facilities. In large facilities, especially in urban areas, there might be several types of units: Alzheimer's units, renal units, or vent units. If your mother has special needs, it will be worth checking out these units. While the other types of specialty units are less common, close to half of the facilities in most areas will have Alzheimer's units.

In general, when you are looking at a specialty unit, the biggest issue is to make sure it really delivers what it promises. Many states do not have specific regulations about specialty units. This leaves it up to you to do your homework on what to expect or not to expect in such a unit.

QUESTIONS TO ASK

ALZHEIMER'S/DEMENTIA CARE

1. Do you have a special program for clients with Alzheimer's or other dementias? What makes it special?
2. What training and/or experience do you and your staff have regarding dementia care?
3. What safety measures do you have in place for wandering behavior?
4. How do you treat nighttime waking? Sundowners Syndrome? Many folks with dementia tend to confuse day and night. Sundowners Syndrome is the tendency to become more agitated during the late afternoon and evening.
5. How do you treat aggressive or combative behavior?
6. What is your approach to chemical and/or physical restraints?
7. Do your clients wear ID or is there some other system in place in case dad wanders away?
8. What activities do you have? Are they dementia specific? Do you take your clients out to community events?
9. Do you have a support group for families? How do you include families in your program?

Hospice Away From Home

As mentioned in Chapter Five, hospice is care specifically designed for the patient with a terminal diagnosis. While hospice agencies usually focus on home hospice care, if needed, the hospice agency can arrange a respite stay in a SNF. The big difference for mom will be that the hospice organization will take over primary responsibility for her care just like they would if she were still at home. The hospice provides nursing, social services, counseling, and pain management to support your mom and your family during the final months. The facility will provide room and board, nursing and other supportive services.

QUESTIONS TO ASK

SKILLED NURSING FACILITIES

1. May I see your last state survey?
2. What is your staffing ratio? This is usually expressed in hours per resident day. To get this number, the total number of working hours per day for nurses and CNAs are divided by the number of residents in a unit. Some states have minimum requirements. Find out what the minimum requirement is in your state and see if the facility meets or exceeds this number.
3. How often will dad have a bath? How often will he be shaved? Is there a beauty/barber shop on-site?
4. Is the facility restraint appropriate? Restraints are appropriate only in very specific medical situations.
5. Who do I talk to when I have questions about dad's care?
6. When are the care plan meetings? If they are scheduled at a time that is not convenient for me, can I ask for a different time?
7. How often will the doctor visit? Some doctors prefer not to visit SNFs. Ask dad's doctor if he will continue to care for dad in the facility or will he transfer to another doctor. Your dad has the right to choose his own doctor.
8. Do you provide transportation for diagnostic tests, dialysis, or other medical related procedures?
9. What therapies are available? Are therapies available on weekends? What notice will I get when therapies end? Can I watch dad's therapy?
10. How does dad get phone calls, mail, etc.? The facility is required to provide a private phone even if there is not a phone in his room.

SKILLED NURSING FACILITIES (Continued)

11. What is the food like? Are snacks available between meals? Try to eat in the dining room. If this is not possible, visit during a meal and ask folks what they think of the food.
12. What happens in an emergency? How quickly will I be notified?
13. What activities are available? Do you take residents to community events?
14. Do you have a social worker? Is counseling available?
15. What are the resident rooms like? Are phones, TVs, or other amenities provided? Can I bring in dad's favorite chair?
16. When can I visit? Most facilities are very open to visitors. They usually just ask that you don't disturb the roommate by late nights or early mornings.
17. Can arrangements be made if dad needs hospice or other special services?
18. Is the facility certified for Medicaid, Medicare, VA, IHS, or other potential funding sources? Do they accept long term care insurance?
19. Are there extra charges for laundry, incontinent supplies, barber/beauty shop, etc.? How do you bill?

HIGHER ACUITY

The hospital is another place where there have been tremendous changes in the last twenty years. Some of these changes include specialty hospitals, technology in diagnosis and treatment, and shorter stays. Surgery does not necessarily mean a hospital admission as many surgeries are now considered outpatient procedures.

If dad has a stroke, the hospital discharge planner may suggest a good place to get him back on his feet is a rehabilitation specialty hospital. Rehab hospitals focus on therapy for folks after traumatic injury or illness. For example, think of the amount of therapy that Christopher Reeves has needed to recuperate to where he is now. This is the level of therapy normally offered at a rehab hospital.

Sometimes, since older people tend to recuperate more slowly, the doctor will suggest moving dad to a skilled facility to begin the recuperation and therapy process and then be transferred to the rehab hospital as his strength increases. It sometimes happens the other way around, too, where a patient starts therapy at the rehab hospital and transfer to the skilled facility as their needs change.

The financial source for most acute care hospital stays will be mom's Medicare with the co-pays covered by her Medi-gap insurance or Medicaid.

SO WHAT'S REALLY THE RIGHT ANSWER?

Now that you have had a quick tour of the types of facilities and organizations available to you, at this point you may be feeling a bit dazed. Deciding what is the right place for mom or dad is really up to you. The answer may change as the care needs change, so even if you feel you have made the right decision now, it may not be the final decision. You may find that mom or dad moves through several levels of care within the same facility or between facilities. That is why, in general, it is a good idea to look for facilities that offer more than just one program.

Before you make any final decisions about facilities or other services it is important to see for yourself what they are really like. If you have the time, visit several facilities of similar kind. Ask some of the questions that are listed with each type of facility and listen carefully to the answers. Beyond these questions, use your own senses. As the saying goes, if it quacks like a duck and walks like a duck it is probably a duck. If a facility just doesn't "feel" right, then it is probably not the right place for your loved one.

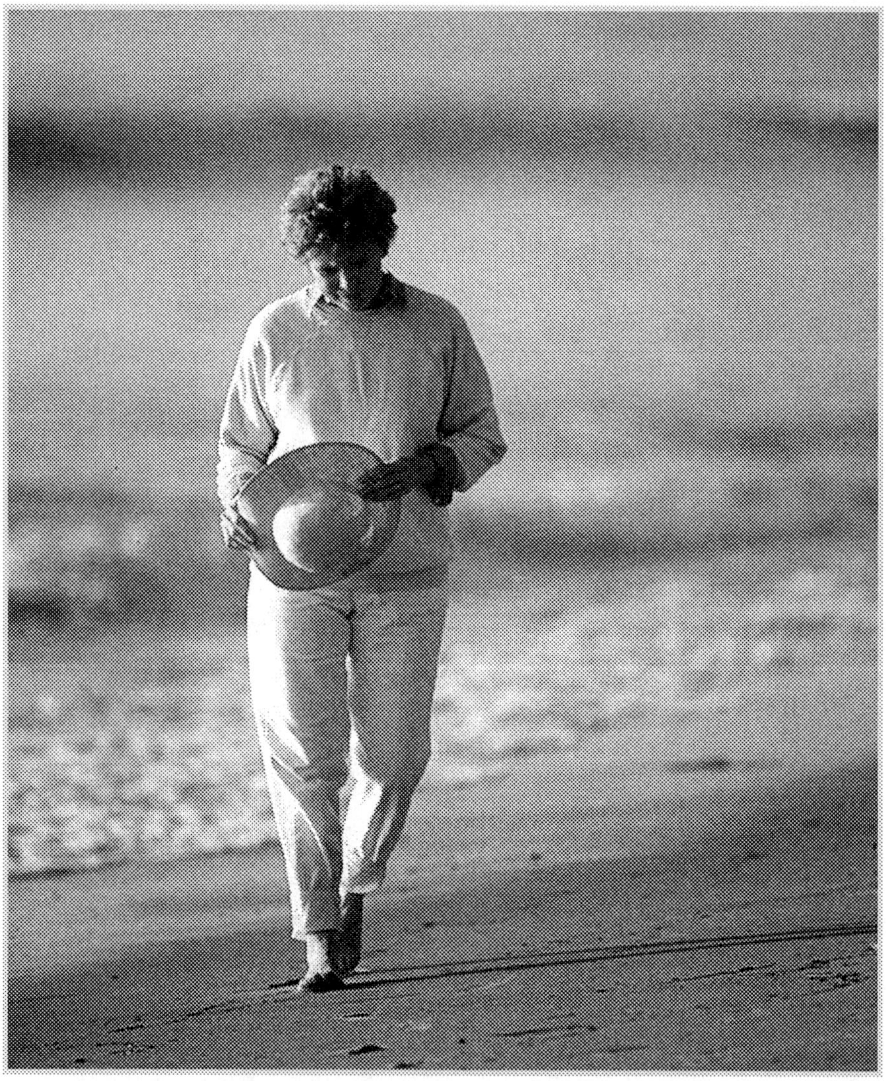

"...Celebrate your life together and try not to fall in the trap of letting the illness become your primary focus..."

CHAPTER NINE:

Coping with Caring

"Wrinkles should merely indicate where smiles have been."
Mark Twain

KNOW WHEN TO SAY "WHEN"

Chapter Two has a list of questions to ask regarding when to intervene for the safety of your parents. Now it is your turn. If you are answering "yes" to more than half of the following list, it is time for someone to intervene with you.

DANGER SIGNS FOR CAREGIVERS

1. Do you have trouble remembering the last time you did something just for fun?
2. When you see other people laughing, do you resent it?
3. Are you beginning to have health problems yourself?
4. Do you feel like you are always tired? Have you not had a good night's sleep in weeks? Or months?
5. When talking to outsiders, do you tend to refer to yourself and dad as "we"?
6. When you are away from mom do you worry constantly about what you will find when you return?
7. Do you think no one else can take care of dad?
8. Have you ever raised your voice in anger or struck the person you are caring for?

DANGER SIGNS FOR CAREGIVERS (Continued)

9. Are your own children and/or spouse starting to resent grandma?

10. Are people who care about you starting to say you need help?

A large portion of this book has dealt with resources to help you in your journey through the Caregiver Zone. If you haven't used any of them yet, now is the time to pick up the phone. Whether it is just to call a friend to go out for lunch or to call the admissions director at a facility, the reality is you need help. It is not a sign of a bad child to ask for the help you need.

By the way, this is also a good time to call those siblings, friends, and others who casually said, "Call me if you need anything." Be realistic about your expectations. Make a list of things that people can do to help and use this as a guide when you call family and friends. For example, brother Joe who lives a thousand miles away probably can't run to the pharmacy for you, but maybe he could pay mom's pharmacy bill. dad's neighbor might not want the responsibility of staying with dad, but he can arrange a Boy Scout troop to clean dad's yard. It is truly amazing what folks are willing to do if they are just told what needs to be done.

WHEN THE WARNING SIGNS ARE IGNORED

Beth is a wonderful daughter. When her widowed mother, Alice, began showing increasing signs of dementia, Beth moved Alice into her own home. As Alice's dementia progressed, Beth took an extended leave from work to care for Alice full time. Beth reasoned that she would only have her mother for a short time and she wanted to be an active part of her mother's last few months. Beth's husband agreed to this plan because he truly loved his mother-in-law.

For a while, despite the dementia, Beth and Alice had a good time. Beth took Alice everyplace: walks in the park, shopping, and to get her hair done once a week. Alice liked to do simple chores like folding laundry and helping with the dishes. Beth cherished her mom's good days and tried to be patient on the bad days.

After about six months, the bad days seemed to increase. Alice repeated the same questions every fifteen minutes. She no longer got the dishes clean and she slopped water all over the kitchen cabinets. Beth found herself spending more time cleaning up after her mother's attempts at helping than it would have taken if she had just washed the dishes herself. Some afternoons, it seemed like all Alice did was pace through the house, rearranging Beth's artfully displayed miniature collection. When Beth took Alice out, Alice would cling to her. Alice didn't even want to get her hair done at the beauty shop any more. One day in the grocery store, Alice wandered away. Beth was embarrassed when she had to ask a stock boy to help locate her mother. Beth's husband complained that Alice did not knock before walking into his bedroom and she sometimes forgot to close the door on her own. Beth got less sleep each night, as Alice was often up several times during the night, turning on lights and opening doors.

Then Alice became incontinent. She actually had an accident on Beth's brand new sofa. Something inside Beth snapped. She grabbed her mother's arm hard enough to leave bruises and pulled Alice down the hall to her bedroom. "You just stay in there while I clean up the mess you made!"

That night, Beth cried all night. How could she have acted like that to her own mother?

Another of the myths of aging is that elder abuse only happens in institutions. Sadly, the National Center on Elder Abuse reports that family members actually account for 61% of substantiated elder abuse reports. Elder abuse is often the result of exhaustion and frustration on the part of the caregiver. Don't let yourself get to that point as you move from the normal stress of caregiving to the distress of total overload.

Of course, not all abuse or neglect is caused by caregiver overload. The horrible reality is that some folks do take advantage of vulnerable older people by abusing them physically or mentally. Con artists, caregivers, or even family members may prey upon older people by taking advantage of them financially.

If you suspect abuse, neglect, or financial exploitation, it is extremely important to report it to your local Adult Protective Services Department. These folks are trained to investigate and stop elder abuse.

Now to some ways to keep yourself balanced as you complete your journey through the Caregiver Zone.

KEEP IT REAL

Muriel's Mom

It was hard not to stare a little at the folks sitting in the wheelchairs. Gray or white hair crowned every head. Hands and feet were twisted by arthritis or missing altogether. So many lines on so many faces. One poor woman looked like half her face had melted and then frozen into a puddle of sagging skin. A little gasp escaped from Muriel's lips.

Heavens, that poor old woman was her mother. For just a second Muriel had forgotten about the Bell's palsy. She had been looking for the other mother—the one who played Barbies and drank Kool-Aid, or at least the one who bustled around organizing church fundraisers and gardening. *Who was this pathetic old woman?*

"Hello, momma."

"Why Muriel, I didn't see you come in."

The pathetic old woman had transformed into momma, again.

From "Wearing Purple" by Judy Castleberry

In the little scene above, Muriel comes to visit her mother in the skilled nursing facility. On her drive to the facility, Muriel reminisces about her mother playing with Muriel as a child. With her memories fresh in her mind, the reality of her mother's present condition is almost too much. However, it takes just a few words to make Muriel's momma real again.

One of the real dangers as a caregiver is losing sight of reality. Some of the things you might be unrealistic about are:

- My mom took care of me as a child so I must take care of her
- My dad made me promise that I would never put him in a nursing home
- No one else can do what I do for mom

- If I do everything right dad will no longer have Alzheimer's or cancer or whatever
- Even though we have never gotten along, I need to move mom into my home to take care of her

Like Muriel, this unrealistic thinking gets in the way of seeing the problem, and if you can't see a problem, you can't solve it. Conversely, if you are so caught up in solving the daily crisis, you are going to miss the moments of sheer joy that come in caregiving.

Relationships and even individual identity tend to get lost in the medication regime, special diets, and linen changes. If you find that happening, maybe it's time to stop for a moment and remember who this person is that you are caring for. Sit down with mom or dad and just visit. Take this time to store up a few memories, forgive old history, and appreciate the person.

That's easy for me to say, right? You were up with dad six times last night, your washing machine seems to be running non-stop, the doctor won't return a phone call, mom has called three times in the last two hours, and your own husband is making ugly comments about another fast food meal. Or maybe you've been reading this book in the waiting room at the hospital. The word "stress" has your picture beside it in the dictionary and now I expect you to do one more thing?

That stress is probably getting in the way of seeing reality, also. So the next few ideas focus on taking care of the stress by getting the problems off your back.

HAVE A BACKUP PLAN

In business, one of the rules is to always have a backup plan for when things go wrong, because they will go wrong. The same principle is true in caregiving. Problems are always going to arise at the worst possible time. This is why so much of this book is devoted to explaining different options. Even if you never use all of these options, knowing what they are and how they work will give you a starting place when things go wrong.

LEARN THE FINE ART OF COMPLAINING

Just like you need to have a general backup plan, you also need to understand your role as your parent's advocate within the system. Most folks in senior care are really trying to provide excellent services. But, in the real world, sometimes problems happen. Understanding how to solve these problems can be a great stress reducer.

Whatever program or facility is providing services, start out by making sure that you really understand what you can expect from the services. Read all of the brochures and pamphlets they hand out. Ask lots of questions before you sign anything, including any complaint procedures.

When something goes wrong, start out by following the complaint procedure. Any facility or agency should have procedures in place for dealing with problems whether the problem is dad's lost comforter or someone being rude to mom. In the real world of senior services, misunderstandings and lost items can happen. Using the official complaint procedure should resolve most issues.

However, if using the complaint procedure doesn't solve the problem, then there are other places to turn. Some suggestions:

- The administrator or manager
- The owner of the agency or facility. Much of senior care is owned by non-profit or for profit corporations. Know who owns the agency or facility that is taking care of mom. Local management should be able to give you a phone number, or look it up on the Internet. If the agency or facility is under the auspices of Area Agency on Aging or another government entity, find out to whom they report at the state or federal level.
- Adult Protective Services. This is the agency responsible for addressing complaints of abuse, exploitation, or neglect of adults. Look in the phone book under state or local government listings.
- Medicare, Medicaid, VA, insurances, and other funding sources have consumer hotlines.

Do not be afraid to complain, but be realistic about complaints. Not every problem can be solved, no matter how far up the chain you go. While it is realistic to complain to a home health agency about an employee who screams at your mom, it is not realistic to expect the agency to bend the Medicare rules about mom's "housebound" status. Likewise, it is realistic to expect a facility to comply with dad's low sodium/low fat/diabetic diet, but it is not realistic to expect them never to serve liver just because your dad doesn't like it. However, they should be able to offer a substitute that your dad will like.

LEARN TO LAUGH

When I worked in facilities, people always asked, "isn't that depressing?" Frankly, one of the main things I found depressing was the automatic assumption that old people are depressing. I've had some pretty good laughs with ninety-year-olds as well as a few one-hundred-year-olds. I've also known a lot of funny morticians.

Anyone who works daily in grim circumstances (firemen, policemen, ER nurses) will tell you that it is the time you are under the most stress that you most need your sense of humor to get you through. Some of the daily things you do as a caregiver can be just plain funny. Look for humor in daily events, read funny stories, and remember that giggling is healing. Learn to laugh with your mom or dad. It will make both of you happier.

BE NICE TO YOURSELF

For folks who are natural caregivers, this is often the hardest rule to follow. It is their nature to always take care of other people first. So if for no other reason than it will keep you ready to serve, take a little time every day to take care of yourself. Use this time to:

- Take a walk
- Go swimming
- Read a book
- Have lunch with someone you can talk to
- Go to worship
- Take a nap
- Dig in your garden
- Do something else that has absolutely nothing to do with caregiving

SPECIAL SUGGESTIONS FOR CAREGIVING SPOUSES

I have been to many fiftieth, sixtieth, and even a few seventy-fifth wedding anniversaries. Often there will be a wedding photo displayed. Looking at the smiling young couple in those photos, it is hard to imagine that they had any idea what was ahead of them. Yet, here they are so many years later, still holding hands. How do you keep that relationship going when you are now the caregiver for that sweet young thing in the picture?

Many of the things we have discussed so far apply to you also: be realistic, have backup plans, know how to complain, and be nice to yourself. Sometimes, though, this is especially hard for spouses. So here are a few additional suggestions for you.

- Do not hesitate to ask your children for help when you need it. Sometimes it is hard to tell the kids that mom is having problems remembering, or you can't clean the house anymore. Most children want to help, but they back off because they believe mom or dad telling them that things are fine. Your children may not be able to solve all the problems, but maybe they can help you find the help you need.

- Keep your spouse at the center of the decisions about his or her care, while realizing the impact on you. Not all decisions are life and death, but many affect the quality of life for both of you. For example, what is the best setting for rehab after a stroke: an acute care rehab hospital, skilled nursing facility, or in your own home with home health? How will this decision affect you? Are you up to the physical demands of caring for your spouse at home? What kind of help will you need? If he goes to a facility, do you have a way of getting there to visit every day?

- Couples who cope well with illness also learn to hold onto what is important and let go of what is not. Whether your spouse is in a facility or at home, you can still share a quiet early morning cup of coffee. Ignore the phone and the housework (or let someone else do it) so that you can have time together. Celebrate your life together and try not to fall into the trap of letting the illness become your primary focus. This is still the man or woman you married all those years ago. Do silly romantic things that have meaning to you. Brighten the room with a bouquet of roses from the bushes you planted in your yard or rent your favorite old movie to watch together.

- Give yourself permission to have some time for yourself. Unless you were a very unusual couple, you probably did not spend every minute of every day of your marriage together, yet many caregivers feel that they must be at their loved one's side at all times.
- Take care of your own health. It is very easy to fall into the trap of neglecting yourself while caring for a spouse. Remind yourself that it will not help your spouse if you become ill, too.

LIVE THIS DAY WITHOUT REGRETS

Wherever you are in the Caregiver Zone, there are probably sources with lots of good advice—maybe even this book. The nice thing about all this advice is that it is yours to take or leave. In the end, what really matters is that mom and dad are able to live out their lives as close to the way they wish as possible.

No one is expecting you to miraculously make your parents twenty-five again, and in perfect health—not even your parents. So put away your rusty old magic wand—it didn't work that well in the first place. Instead, give yourself permission to just concentrate on what needs to be done today. After all, those of us in senior care know that today is sometimes all you get. So make today as good a day as possible and you won't have any regrets tomorrow.

FINAL THOUGHTS

Recently, I was having a conversation with an adult daughter. Some difficult decisions had to be made regarding care. The daughter said, "This is so hard. Why can't it be easier?"

Caregiving is not an easy role. It means dealing with things that many of us would choose not to deal with if we had another option. Caregiving, like greatness, is sometimes just thrust upon us when we really aren't ready.

Over the years, I have known some truly wonderful families. I have watched in awe as they gracefully coped with the symptoms of Alzheimer's, cancer, and many other conditions. It wasn't that their life was easier or they had more resources. What seemed to make the difference was the approach they took to caregiving. They realized that old age is just as much a part of life as growing up and that most of us will someday be old ourselves. They understand the beauty in wrinkles and gray hair when they are attached to someone they love.

APPENDICES

APPENDIX A: Checklists and Tables

The numerous checklists and tables used in this book are also available on our website. This can be printed and used as a workbook as you travel through The Caregiver Zone.
Go to http://www.TheCaregiverZone.com\forms.

The Last Checklist: COORDINATING CARE

As you are arranging care for your parents, there are a few basics that will need to be addressed in any setting. Often new caregivers overlook some of these basics or underestimate the cost in time or dollars. This final checklist is intended to help you think through what is really involved in providing care.

NEEDS	ASSISTANCE NEEDED	TIME & FREQUENCY	PROVIDER	COST
Activities of Daily Living				
Bathing Baths/Showers	Independent Reminders Help in/out of tub/shower Total assistance Bed baths			
Dressing	Independent Assistance			
Brushing Teeth/ Washing Face/etc.	Independent Assistance			
Men - Shaving	Independent Assistance			

NEEDS	ASSISTANCE NEEDED	TIME & FREQUENCY	PROVIDER	COST
Activities of Daily Living				
Hair Care Beauty/ Barber Shop Washing/brushing	Independent Assistance			
Walking	Independent Assistance			
*Wheelchair transfers	Independent Assistance			
Food				
Shopping				
Preparing Meals		Breakfast Lunch Dinner		
Special Diet:				
Eating		Independent Needs food cut Needs to be fed		
Medications				
Delivery/Pickup				
Taking Medication		Independent Pill Box Reminders Administred		

NEEDS	ASSISTANCE NEEDED	TIME & FREQUENCY	PROVIDER	COST
Medical Care				
Oxygen/ Inhalation Treatments				
Dressings/ Bandages				
Dialysis				
Therapies				
Other				
Household				
Daily Cleaning				
Weekly Cleaning				
Laundry				
Transportation/ Errands				
Household/Yard Maintenance				

APPENDIX B: Friends and Resources

National Resources

Aging Information

Administration on Aging
www.aoa.gov
(877) 696-6775

AARP
www.aarp.org
(888) 687-2277

National Area Agencies on Aging
www.4na.org
(800) 677-1116

National Institute on Aging
www.nia.nih.gov
(301) 496-1752

Caregiver Support & Information

Children of Aging Parents
www.caps4caregivers.org
(800) 227-7294

Eldercare Locator
www.eldercare.gov/eldercare/public/home.asp

Family Caregiver Alliance
www.caregiver.org
(800) 445-8106

National Center on Elder Abuse
www.elderabusecenter.org
(202) 898-2586

Disease-Specific Information & Support

Alzheimer's Association
www.alz.org
(800) 272-3900

Alzheimer's Disease Education & Referral Center
www.alzheimer.org
(800) 438-4380

American Parkinson Disease Association
www.apdaparkinson.org
(800) 400-2732

Arthritis Foundation
www.arthritis.org
(800) 283-7800

Disease-Specific Information & Support (continued)

American Diabetes Association
www.diabetes.org
(800) 342-2383

American Heart Association
www.americanheart.org
(800) 242-8721

Financial and Legal Issues

Center for Medicare and Medicaid
www.cms.hhs.gov
(877) 267-2323

National Academy of Elder Law Attorneys
www.naela.org
(520) 881-4005

Medicare
www.medicare.gov
1-800-medicare

Professional, Service, & Trade Organizations

American Health Care Association
www.ahca.org
(202) 842-4444

National Association for Home Care
www.nahc.org
(202) 547-7424

American Association of Homes and Services for the Aging
www.aahsa.org
(202) 783-2242

National Association of Professional Geriatric Care Managers
www.caremanager.org
(520) 881-8008

Meals on Wheels
www.mowaa.org
(703) 548-5558

National Private Duty Association
www.privatedutyhomecare.org
(317) 844-7105

Local Resources

Your best resource for locating services locally is your phone book.

Yellow Pages Headings

Assisted Living Facilities
Home Health Agencies
Hospice
Hospitals
Nursing Homes
Medical Alarms and Monitoring
Rehabilitation Hospitals and Services
Senior Citizen Services

Government Pages

Federal Government

- Health & Human Services
- Social Security Administration
- Veterans Affairs

State Government

(May vary in your area)

- Area Agency on Aging
- Adult Protective Services
- Children, Youth, and Families
- Commission for the Blind
- Health Department
- Human Services
- Income Support Division
- Office of Senior Affairs
- Welfare Department

City Government

- Adult Protective Services
- Health Department
- Human Services

APPENDIX C: Learning the Lingo

Activities of Daily Living (ADL). Self care and related tasks that a person does each day: bathing, dressing, grooming, eating, walking, toileting, etc.

Acute. Sudden and/or short term severe condition. Also refers to a high level of care such as an acute care hospital.

Adult Day Care. Congregate day care for adults including meals and structured activities. Some adult day care programs also offer transportation and healthcare.

Advance Directives. A document that directs healthcare and other care for an individual.

Alzheimer's Disease. A progressive and irreversible organic disease causing progressive memory loss, eventually physical deterioration, and death.

Ambulate. Walk.

Aphasia. Loss of the ability to talk and/or understand language.

Care Management. Usually contracted individually (occasionally through insurance), this program is intended to coordinate all services provided to an individual including medical, housing, non-medical care, etc.

Care Plan. A written plan of care and services provided to a person by a long term care facility, home health agency, or other service. The care plan should include needs, goals, methods to achieve the goals, and a time frame for accomplishing the goals.

Case Management. Under certain government programs or insurances, this service is intended to coordinate medical care and services for an individual.

Certificate of Medical Necessity. A document required by Medicare and insurances that is signed by the doctor to certify that the patient needs certain types of durable medical equipment.

Certified Nursing Assistant (CNA). An individual who has attended a training course and passed the applicable written and skills test. CNAs provide personal care such as bathing, dressing, grooming, and assistance with eating, transfers to bed and wheelchair, etc. CNAs practice in long term care facilities, home health agencies, hospices, and hospitals.

Chronic. As opposed to acute, this is a condition that will continue for a long time, possibly for life.

Cognitive Impairment. Refers to a loss of mental ability, including difficulty with short and/or long term memory.

Companion Care. Non-medical services such as preparing meals, housekeeping, laundry, errands and transportation, friendly visiting, grooming, and safety supervision.

Conservator. A person appointed by the court to act as the legal representative of a person who is unable to handle their own affairs due to mental or physical limitations.

Decubitis. Also called a bed sore or pressure ulcer, this is when the skin breaks down into a sore because of pressure on fragile skin. Decubitis are often caused by lack of movement, poor fluid intake, incontinence, and fragile skin due to aging and/or disease.

Dementia. Loss of memory and/or cognitive ability. Alzheimer's is the most prevalent cause of dementia.

Diagnostic Related Groups (DRGs). A coding system that Medicare uses to determine payments to hospitals.

Durable Medical Equipment (DME). Equipment such as wheelchairs, walkers, hospital beds, and elevated commodes.

Durable Medical Power of Attorney. A document signed by an individual to give another person the power to make health care decisions if he is unable to.

Edema. When fluid collects in the tissues causing swelling.

Emergency Response System. An electronic devise for the home that summons assistance in an emergency. Usually consists of a button that the individual wears on the wrist or a pendant that uses the phone to call emergency dispatch.

Fiscal Intermediary. Under Medicare, this is the private insurance company contracted to handle claims.

Incompetent. Legally, this means that a court has found a person unable to handle their own financial and legal affairs.

Incontinent. Unable to control bowel and/or bladder functions.

Minimum Data Set (MDS). A broad based assessment of each patient in a Medicare and Medicaid certified long term care facility. Medicare payment (and in some states Medicaid payment) is based upon each patient's rating. The assessment includes medical, physical, social, dietary, activities, and other information.

Medically Necessary. The concept that a physician must determine if a certain treatment, service, or procedure is necessary for medical care before an insurance will pay for it.

Ombudsman. A program (usually through the Area Agency on Aging) that provides volunteers to visit and advocate for the rights of residents in long term care facilities, assisted living facilities, or other senior services.

Provider. An agency, institution, or other services that provides care, services or equipment.

Resident. The term, similar to patient or client, used to describe someone living in long term care.

Resident Assistant (RA). The workers in assisted living facilities that provide personal care services. In most states, they are not certified as CNAs.

Respite Care. Short term care by another provider to give relief to the primary caregiver. This may include companion care, hospice, long term care facility, or other provider.

Sub-acute Care. The level of care usually following an acute illness when acute care is no longer needed, but extensive therapy, skilled nursing, and other services are required. Sub-acute units may be in an acute care hospital or long term care facility.